AfterShock

"Anyone with a scary diagnosis would do him/herself a favo[...] without delay. *AfterShock* is wise, sensitive, practical, reada[...] extreme."
　　　　　　　　　　—Betty Rollin, author of *First, You Cry* and *Here's the Bright Side*

"This is an extraordinary guide based on solid research and depth of expertise. It is infused with clarity, wit, wisdom, compassion, and most of all, hope."
　　　　　　　　　　—Vartan Gregorian, President, Carnegie Corporation of New York

"Each of us, or one of our loved ones, is likely to receive a diagnosis of devastating illness. That is why this perceptive, comforting, and practical book belongs on every family's shelf."
　　—Joseph A. Califano Jr., Chairman and President, the National Center on Addiction and Substance Abuse (CASA) at Columbia University, and former U.S. Secretary of Health, Education and Welfare, 1977–1979

"In this period of bewildering complexity in our fragmented health system, Jessie Gruman's book is a quiet, reassuring refuge from the challenge of receiving shocking medical news—empowering to the patient and to his/her family, helping them to become active participants in the planning and the delivery of their health care and health maintenance. *AfterShock* is an invaluable medical resource and supportive companion."
　　—Louis W. Sullivan, M.D., President Emeritus, Morehouse School of Medicine, and U.S. Secretary of Health and Human Services, 1989–1993

"This is a book about life. The poignant stories attest to the enduring value of friends and family—as well as medical professionals—in helping find a path through the painful first shock and wrenching turmoil of a life-changing diagnosis. Everyone can benefit from this book. Don't wait until you think you need it. Read it now."
　　—Mary O'Neil Mundinger, Dr.P.H., R.N., Dean and Centennial Professor in Health Policy, Columbia University School of Nursing

"When someone close to you is diagnosed with a serious illness, do them a big favor—give them this book. Dr. Gruman has written a compelling and comprehensive guide to making use of the best available evidence to respond to a bad diagnosis."　　　　　　　　　　**—John W. Rowe, M.D.**, Executive Chairman, Aetna

"Jessie Gruman knows of what she speaks. If you or a loved one has received a devastating diagnosis, *AfterShock* sympathetically lays out what to do and how to do it. Gruman's book is clear, concise, wide-ranging, elegantly composed, richly illustrated by personal reflections, deeply informed, and highly practical. This is a work I will want to share with family and friends."
　　　　　　　　　　—Harvey V. Fineberg, M.D., Ph.D., President, Institute of Medicine

"For patients and families faced with bad diagnostic news, it would be hard to find a more useful and dependable support. Jessie Gruman is wise, practical, and authoritative—and she's been there."
　　　　　　　　　　—Jeremiah Barondess, M.D., President, New York Academy of Medicine

"If someone you love has ever had a frightening diagnosis, they surely could have used Jessie Gruman's book. By assuring you that your initial state of shock is normal, then by guiding you through the ways to make the tough choices, *AfterShock* helps restore the sense of control you probably lost. A how-to on getting the best care, the book is both reassuring and empowering."

—**Lesley Stahl**, correspondent on *60 Minutes*, CBS

"No doctor can tell you everything you need to know about how to respond to a devastating diagnosis. *AfterShock* can help you make good choices about all the elements of your new and challenging situation. Jessie Gruman is a great friend of seriously ill patients. If you let her help you—she will."

—**David Nathan, M.D.**, President Emeritus, Dana-Farber Cancer Institute

"The discovery of a medical problem causes a crisis not only for the patient but also for the family. The author, having been through these unsettling problems several times and having shown remarkable resilience, lays out practical suggestions on what to do and also how to relieve the stress."

—**Aaron T. Beck, M.D.**, University Professor of Psychiatry, University of Pennsylvania, and Lasker Award recipient

"This is a splendid example of turning one's recurrent frightening situation into a positive gift for others. I think the book will be most helpful to people who seek more information. They will be able to return to the book repeatedly as their need for different information and their readiness to use it change as they adapt to their devastating diagnosis. This book, like its characterization of many nurses, is 'pure gold.' "

—**Martha N. Hill, Ph.D., R.N.**, Dean, Johns Hopkins University School of Nursing

"The medical community owes Dr. Gruman a huge thanks for writing this courageous book. Anyone confronting some of the frightening diseases that it is our great misfortune to suffer can be comforted and guided by this wonderful volume."

—**Kenneth L. Davis, M.D.**, President and CEO, Mount Sinai Medical Center

"Reading this gorgeously written book is both an emotional and intellectual experience. It is a 'must have' for anyone touched by a devastating illness either directly or through a loved one. Any health professional not deeply moved by the contents should find another line of work."

—**Claire Fagin, Ph.D., R.N.**, Dean Emerita, University of Pennsylvania School of Nursing

"After the shock of a devastating diagnosis comes the 'aftershock,' when a person must learn the topography of a strange and frightening terrain. Written with unpretentious authority, *AfterShock* is a humane and immensely important book about coping with a catastrophic illness."

—**Robert M. Butler, M.D.**, President and CEO, International Longevity Center, USA

"*AfterShock* is an amazing guide for the overwhelmed person or family member asking 'What do I do next?' It is filled with practical advice which is mixed—in a most pleasantly readable style—with the observations of someone who has 'been there, done that' but who also knows the psychological terrain of illness. Gruman recognized the gap in information for this period and has filled it beautifully."

—**Jimmie C. Holland, M.D.**, Department of Psychiatry and Behavioral Sciences, Memorial Sloan-Kettering Cancer Center

AfterShock

What to Do When the Doctor Gives You
—or Someone You Love—
a Devastating Diagnosis

Jessie Gruman, Ph.D.

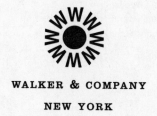

WALKER & COMPANY

NEW YORK

Published by Walker Publishing Company, Inc., New York
Distributed to the trade by Holtzbrinck Publishers

All papers used by Walker & Company are natural,
recyclable products made from wood grown in
well-managed forests. The manufacturing processes conform
to the environmental regulations of the country of origin.

Library of Congress Cataloging-in-Publication Data
has been applied for.

ISBN-10: 0-8027-1502-8
ISBN-13: 978-0-8027-1502-9

Visit Walker & Company's Web site at
www.walkerbooks.com

First U.S. edition 2007

1 3 5 7 9 10 8 6 4 2

Typeset by Westchester Book Group
Printed in the United States of America by
Quebecor World Fairfield

THIS BOOK IS DEDICATED to the hundreds of individuals with experience in responding to a devastating diagnosis whose stories are reflected here. Having faced such diagnoses four times, I know that it is not an easy or welcome task to be asked to recall this painful time—to describe one's despair, confusion, or lack of preparation to meet the challenge of a serious threat to one's life. Those who talked with me were not only willing to do this, but were generous to a fault. They told not only of their panic but also how they coped; not only of their setbacks and disappointments, but also of the things they learned and the ways they maintained their dignity and autonomy.

Each of them was willing to relive their own response to bad medical news in the hope that their hard-won lessons might ease the suffering of others.

I am grateful for their wisdom and am honored by their trust in me to transmit their stories in a book that may be useful for you.

INTRODUCTION

When I think about what it was like getting a devastating diagnosis, I have a picture of these two full grocery carts coming toward each other at top speed. They collide at full force and then in slow motion, all the vegetables, the cantaloupe, the eggs, the apples, and the bread go flying into the air. And I'm just watching—helpless to prevent the collision, helpless to save the groceries. But eventually, slowly they fall: the eggs shatter, the bread is smashed—it is such a mess.

That is what it was like for me hearing that I have a disease that will rob me of my independence—and maybe my life—within the year. Time seemed to stop and it was as though I was looking through a window: watching the doctors talking, my wife responding, people on the street going about their lives. I was frozen. Later—the next day, I think—what this meant began to sink in: the end of my future, the end of our plans.

And then my heart broke.

Eli, 28—banker

THIS IS A BOOK ABOUT what you must do to take care of yourself while your heart is breaking.

Receiving bad health news sparks great personal upheaval. Some people rage against the unfairness, others wither from sadness. Some people lose their faith, others find it. Some are torn between their fear of pain and their fear of death. Families are wracked by the threat of loss. It is a time when nothing is certain and the future looks dark.

And in the midst of this anguish, each one of us, irrespective of diagnosis—cancer, ALS, HIV/AIDS, Alzheimer's disease, multiple sclerosis—will by necessity undertake a number of tasks to care for ourselves that we have probably never done before but that can have an important impact on the lives of everyone involved.

We will:

- Respond to the shock

- Learn about the condition and its treatments

- Decide whether to involve others

- Find the right doctors and hospitals

- Get timely medical appointments

- Seek other opinions about what is wrong and what to do about it

- Manage our work lives

- Pay for care

- Find relief

- Take the next steps

AfterShock provides practical guidance about how you and your loved ones might approach these tasks while you are in shock about your diagnosis and uncertain about how to respond to it.

Having surveyed the research literature on each of these tasks, I have assembled tips to guide you through them. There are interviews with scores of people from all walks of life who have taken on these tasks—as patients, as family members, and as friends. Also included are interviews with professionals who are involved with people just after they are diagnosed: doctors, nurses, clergy, social workers, psychiatrists, psychologists, as well as health-plan administrators, clinic staff, and employers.

I wrote this book in the hope that this information, these insights, and these experiences will provide its readers with a sense of their choices without making them feel overwhelmed by what they must learn and do.

My Perspective Is Both Personal and Professional

I am no stranger to life-altering diagnoses.

Four times I have been diagnosed with life-threatening conditions. Each time the news stopped me cold, landing me in the hospital, forcing me to rearrange my schedule and responsibilities while my body was battered by drugs and surgery, and I desperately tried to figure out how to regain my strength.

Three times the diagnosis involved different kinds of cancer and once a dangerous heart condition. All of them were unexpected. All were unwelcome. All of them disrupted my plans.

When the health crisis was resolved, I returned—months or years later—to some variant of the life I had been leading before. At the time of my most recent diagnosis, I was writing another book—on what the public needs to know about the potential and limitations of health research—when my doctor scheduled me for a routine colonoscopy in honor of my fiftieth birthday. Since then, a large part of my colon and I have gone our separate ways, and I wrote this book instead.

Whenever I have received a serious diagnosis, I was stunned, then anguished as I recounted my diagnosis to my family, explaining to them something I didn't fully understand and trying to reassure them while I was quaking at the prospect of what was to come.

Each time I have stood in awe of how much energy it takes to get from the bad news to actually starting on the return path to health: figuring out whether my diagnosis was right and what course of treatment to take—slogging through the tests, searching the Internet, getting to know all the new doctors and their receptionists, arranging for coverage by my insurance, comforting my parents—all while feeling somewhere between extremely anxious and downright terrible.

I have learned much about this immediate postdiagnosis period from my own experiences and from the many others I have encountered over the years who have gone through these same anguished days.

I bring years of professional experience to this challenge.

I have spent the past two decades in the private, nonprofit, and public sectors at AT&T, the American Cancer Society, and the National Cancer Institute, working to help people use credible scientific information in their health decisions. For the past fifteen years, I have directed the Center for the Advancement of Health, a nonpartisan Washington-based organization whose mission is to improve health by promoting the translation of health research into information that individuals can use to make good decisions about their health and health care.

While I have had the bad luck of having these serious health challenges, I have also had the good luck to be able to gather information and share it with others who have just received a serious diagnosis. My training gave me the technical background and my professional position gave me the access to health-care providers, staff, and administrators who have expertise and concern about this time in people's lives.

In writing this book, I interviewed more than 250 people: patients, family members, nurses, doctors, health plan administrators, managers of busy practices and nonprofit leaders. Many of them allowed me to question them only because they accepted me as a colleague, either because of my professional background or because of our common experience of responding to a devastating diagnosis.

Along with this personal experience and background in biomedical, behavioral, and social science, I bring a strong conviction that this book is needed and that my perspective and the experiences of others will help those who find themselves scrambling for answers after the shock of the diagnosis of a life-altering condition.

I am a reluctant consumer.

It is popular in health policy circles to call people who use health-care services "health-care consumers." I know lots of people who are superb consumers. They decide to buy a new camera and then dive into the task of fully exploring every aspect of the camera they want. They know which model has which functions; they know which manufacturers have better service records. They have price shopped and know exactly what the trade-offs are for cost and quality. These people are great to talk to if you want to buy a camera.

I always try to talk to them because I am not like this. I want someone to say, "Here is the perfect camera for you, and look! It's on sale!"

I am especially like this when I have been given a new and really bad diagnosis. Then I want someone to say, "Here is what we are going to do to fix this and you will be completely cured in a couple weeks. Plus, everything will be covered by your insurance!"

But this hasn't happened. Each time I have received a serious diagnosis, I had no idea what I needed or wanted. The choices unfolded over time. Yet increasingly, I have had to force myself to act like a consumer with regard to my health care—because there is so much uncertainty about what's wrong and so many options for what might be done about it; because no one else seems to be taking charge; and because I need to understand what is going on since the decisions I must make are going to affect how I live the rest of my life.

It's a funny thing: Years ago when medical knowledge was far less advanced, everything seemed far more certain. Doctors pretty much told us what treatment we were going to get and that was it. For some people this hasn't changed: we get a diagnosis and it is, as Laura, an administrator, described it, "as though I got on the train and the train kept going," passed from primary care doctor to a specialist who orders a specific course of treatment. All the patient does is show up.

For a variety of reasons, however, this is no longer the norm. A cultural change has taken place in the United States in recent decades. Whether as a reaction to the perceived excesses of managed care or out of a greater understanding of the gaps in knowledge about disease, people are deferring less to medical authority. The pace of discovery about health has accelerated; so much more is now known. And many doctors are reluctant to take charge the way they used to. Now there are treatment choices—decisions that only we can make because they will affect whether we can walk or drive or live out our days drugged and in pain. Many of us are likely to have a number of specialists working on different aspects of our care. Our care may be influenced by our geographic location and insurance coverage.

The upshot is that we have to act as consumers whether we like it or not.

This book is for both highly motivated and reluctant consumers. For motivated people, it illuminates the tasks that need to be done immediately after a diagnosis and gives you avenues to explore for more in-depth information. And for those who are reluctant, it explains why and how to do some very basic things that will help you figure out what decisions you must make so you can take the first few steps forward after hearing the bad news.

My Point of View

AfterShock is not a bossy book. My aim is to give you a manage-able number of good choices from among the millions that are available. In doing so, I have made many judgments about what to include and what to leave out. My judgments are guided by these assumptions:

Receiving a life-altering diagnosis can cause tremendous emotional and spiri-tual upheaval but you still have to figure out the mundane details of getting the care you need and arranging your life to accommodate this new reality. This book focuses specifically on the practical aspects of what you have to do after you get a serious diagnosis, though it is written with an appreciation of the emotional turmoil you may feel.

People have the right to understand what is going on in their body, be given a realistic sense of how treatment might affect it, and the responsibility to make decisions informed by that knowledge. We are, after all, the ones who will live with the consequences of our choices.

Science gives us the best shot at certainty about how the body works and thus gives us the best guidance about the onset, progression, and treatment of disease. Science, while imperfect, offers an objective, systematic approach that can correct its own errors. I put my faith in this approach over anecdotes as the basis of disease treatment any day.

Medicine is part science and part art. Doctors, nurses, and other health professionals have training and experience that gives them the ability to tailor population–based research and risk ratios to one person's situation. While some are better at this than others, health professionals are key to capturing the full value of hard–won sci-entific knowledge in finding the right approach to treating you.

There are many ways to find the care you need immediately after a diagnosis, even though you are under considerable stress. The experiences of how others figured this out can increase your confidence that you are heading in the right direction and reduce some of the uncertainty you feel as you make your way forward.

Most people are doing the best they can at any given time. This includes doctors and nurses and hospital administrators and the people who answer the phones at your health plan provider. But there are competing interests that may interfere. Sometimes those interests are a sick kid at home, sometimes they are the demands of too much work in too little time, and sometimes they are things like the need to make payroll or serve shareholder interests. This book is not a critique of health care in the United States. Rather, it provides guidance about how to cautiously negotiate a confusing, complicated network of institutions and services.

While serious illness can shatter your sense of a well-ordered life, it does not mean that the strength and wisdom of your years are irrelevant to the challenge you face. No matter what your condition, you have choices. They aren't always the choices you would like, and sometimes it may feel like you are unprepared to weigh all the options and make the right decision. But you know yourself. You know what you need to be comfortable, and you know generally what you want. The challenge will be to understand and make those choices with confidence that they are the right ones for you.

How to Use this Book

Every time I have received bad health news, I have felt like a healthy person who has been accidentally drop-kicked into a foreign country: I don't know the language, the culture is unfamiliar, I have no idea what is expected of me, I have no map, and I desperately want to find my way home.

This is a guidebook to help you find your way through these first few weeks. It provides information to help you avoid getting lost and to feel confident that you are doing what you can to resolve this crisis with as few wrong turns as possible.

It was written to be read by people who are having a hard time concentrating. Most people are overwhelmed by the amount of information they have to take in during the time immediately after a devastating diagnosis. You need to learn about your disease and its treatment.

But you are more than your prostate gland or retina or nerve endings. Understanding what has gone wrong in your body and what that means is important, but it is only a small part of what you need to know to get through this time. Figuring out how to manage your family life, getting the tests, and finding the doctors to treat you—while fending off work demands and worrying about how to pay for this unforeseen emergency—require that you take in and act on a lot of information in a short time.

AfterShock divides the things you need to do during this period into manageable tasks.

This book has no plot that you need to follow from start to finish. Your experience with this diagnosis will unfold in a way that is unique to you. Use the table of contents or the index to find the parts about what you are facing today; maybe read a little about what you think is going to happen next. The day after tomorrow, take another look: you will have moved on to another set of questions.

The book is organized to provide three levels of information on each of the subjects almost all people must address when they receive a devastating diagnosis.

First Level: Each chapter opens with an aim. Each time I received a devastating diagnosis I had the same experience: my mind would swing back and forth between complete obsession with details—how to get this test result to that doctor by Tuesday, for example—and the black hole of grief and fear of the future. I couldn't concentrate on anything long enough to feel like I was making any progress.

To help you keep your focus on you where you want to end up as you take on these tasks, each chapter begins with a goal statement—a North Star–like navigation aid that orients you to what you are trying to do at this stage.

So, for example, your aim in finding the right physician is to "find doctors who treat you with respect, who listen and respond to your concerns, in whose expertise you have confidence and whom you trust to do their best for you." Should you start to feel frustrated in your search for a doctor you can work with—you think yours is smart but you really dislike his manner, for example—go back to that orienting statement. Are you taking actions in line with that aim or are you getting bogged down in details? Are you obsessing about his or her insensitivity and not taking steps to find a specialist who is more compatible?

Second Level: Each chapter contains information that will help you make decisions about what to do. The chapters are made up of short sections, each of which addresses a question about some aspect of the task you are taking on. The answers include both evidence-based information and the voices of individuals who approached the task at hand. Not only will you read about why you might seek additional opinions, for example, but you will also hear from others— including me—about how we worried about offending our doctor, where to find other opinions, and how we resolved these concerns.

Third Level: Appendices describe how and where to find the information, professionals, and organizations described in the chapters. Some appendices stand on their own as "how-to" assistance, so at some point, you may want to leaf through them to see if there is something you missed.

Not everyone who receives a serious diagnosis needs this book.

It is written for people who are feeling both desperate about their future and uncertain about how best to approach the unfamiliar challenges ahead. If you are too upset to figure out what questions you should ask your doctor, or your mind is racing as you try to calculate the financial impact of this diagnosis on your family, or you can't focus your attention sufficiently to narrow a Google search of your disease that has yielded 8 million hits, you need pretty specific help. I have tried to offer such help here.

CHAPTER 1

In Shock

Your aim during the first few days is to absorb the news as best you can and to weather the storm of your own emotions and the responses of those who love you.

The doctor said "I'm sorry to have to tell you this terrible news." And he told me. Then he said, "You can't go to work. You can't go to conferences. You must take care of this immediately."

It took all my strength not to break. I had to concentrate all my energy on keeping my legs underneath me. I remember trying to find my way to the exit of the hospital and wobbling—"Just stay upright!" I told each leg. Then I came across some painted signs on the floor that showed the way to the door and I followed them out into the rainy night.

Lucia, 57—government minister

I'm Stunned...

FOR THE FIRST FORTY-EIGHT HOURS after receiving a devastating diagnosis, most people don't feel they have many choices. They are doing the best they can just to take in the news.

There is nothing in my experience or in the experiences of those I interviewed that can take away the distress you feel. But there may be small things—reassurance that you are not going crazy, things you might forget to do because you are so distracted—that will anchor you and help you feel less disoriented.

The purpose of this chapter is to provide an explanation of how shocking news affects your body and mind, and to describe common responses. It includes recommendations of health-care professionals and clergy with expertise in helping people during this time; recounts a range of experiences of people and their loved ones; and examines some common reactions where people frequently get stuck.

And it provides simple, commonsense advice about getting through these first hours.

What Is Happening to Me?

No doubt you have heard about people who perform superhuman feats of strength and courage after a car accident, such as a father lifting a truck off the leg of his son. The rush of adrenaline and the focused attention that make this possible are characteristics of our reaction to danger. This is a powerful and primitive physical response to threat.

When you receive a diagnosis that radically alters your sense of the future, you may have this reaction. Your life *is* in danger. You may experience physical and mental effects that are similar to those of the father whose son is trapped, or similar to those of the son—you are focused on the danger your diagnosis poses to your own life and to the lives of those you love and who depend on you:

- Your thoughts may be racing or may be stuck on one thing.

- You may cry, rage, or withdraw from your friends and family.

- You may be physically restless or may feel drained of energy.

Typical mental and physical reactions to threat are listed more fully later in this chapter. There are many of them and you will probably have only a few of them. The good part is that most of them will subside within a few hours or at most, a couple of days, as you realize that the danger is not imminent *today* and as you begin to fill in the blanks about what your diagnosis means and to plan to manage the danger your diagnosis poses to your future.

THE RANGE OF COMMON RESPONSES
People vary widely in the way they respond to the shock of bad medical news. Some find God. Some lose faith. Denial, rage,

depression, sadness, bargaining, and guilt are all common responses. While a few of us become coldly rational problem-solvers,
many of us experience a tumbling rush of mental and physical
responses. There is no "normal."

It is important to know about the range of common reactions
because:

- You may confuse signs of shock with symptoms of your
  condition, which can be frightening.

- You need to be able to distinguish between a response
  that will soon subside on its own and one for which it
  would be good to seek help.

- Anyone who is close to the person with the serious diagnosis may have similar reactions; this often happens with
  spouses and family members. And even if they are not
  having a strong reaction, they need to know about the
  common range of responses in order to understand how
  they can help you.

Here is a list of ways people often respond to shocking news. No
one experiences them all but some of them will be familiar to
anyone who has experienced a sudden life-threatening event.

Typical *emotional responses* to shocking news are:

Sadness
Despair
Irritation
Rage
Apathy
Guilt
Shame
Giddiness
Mood swings
Withdrawal

Cognitive responses include:

Confusion
Forgetfulness

Difficulty in concentrating
Agitation
Rigid thinking/difficulty incorporating new knowledge
Intrusive or repetitive thoughts

Common *physical* responses are:

Crying
Appetite disruption
Pain: headache, stomachache
Heightened sensitivity to normal physical complaints
Lethargy
Agitation and hyperactivity
Sleep disturbances

The fact that these responses are common doesn't mean that they are to be dismissed as nothing. Any one of these responses is distressing. The important thing to remember is that these are all signs that your body and mind are mobilized to protect you.

WHAT HAVE OTHERS FOUND HELPFUL IN CALMING DOWN?

People vary widely in their desire to tell others immediately, to see people during the first few days after a diagnosis, and to allow others to comfort and reassure them.

Immediately following my most recent diagnosis, I couldn't talk to anyone: it was the only thing I thought I had to talk about and I couldn't do that without crying, so I asked my husband to tell my family members and a few friends. For the two days, I mostly alternated between feeling numb and visiting and revisiting every worst-case scenario about my future that my imagination could conjure. I couldn't read, wasn't interested in looking up my condition on the Web, couldn't concentrate, couldn't find comfort or distraction anywhere. I wanted to jump out of my skin. I ached for more information about my own situation—my own pathology reports—not about the condition in general. I just needed to know enough to make some decisions. But I had to wait for the test results to come back before I saw the doctor again, and those thirty-six hours were excruciating.

What was most helpful? Petting the pets—those innocent, busy little fellows. And doing things I knew were good for me that would take a specific amount of time: Walk to the store and back. Pay bills. I was filling the time until I could find out what was going to happen to me.

I asked the people I interviewed what helped them get through the first forty-eight hours. Here are some of the things they said:

> I called my minister—whom I don't really know that well (I am not very religious). I told him this had just happened and I was in such despair. He came over that evening and I remember nothing of what he said. But I do remember that somehow his visit left me feeling like I was ready to face whatever came next.
>
> Ben, 30—graduate student

> My partner and I came home from the hospital and immediately went online and frantically searched out everything about [her] condition. We are both health professionals and researchers, so I guess this was a natural first response. After about an hour, we stopped. We couldn't take in what we were reading. We just couldn't make sense of it. We didn't know enough about the specifics of her condition. Everything we read about terrified us. So we just quit. In hindsight, I think we felt like we had fulfilled our expectations that we are sensible consumers.
>
> Charlotte, 45—professor

> My friend, whom I help with her treatment—I am her treatment buddy—was so angry when she was diagnosed that she went home and shut herself in her apartment for twenty-four hours: no phone calls, didn't answer the door. Later she said she was overcome with rage and that she spent [those] twenty-four hours pounding the pillow and the walls, screaming and crying and shouting about the unfairness of this disease happening to her. She said that this was something she needed to do for herself and on her own. This was *her* life, *her* diagnosis, *her* death and she wasn't ready to share this yet, even with her parents or her close friends.
>
> Maya, 36—artist

We found it too exhausting and upsetting to call and tell all our family members about the news of my wife's diagnosis of pancreatic cancer. We felt like we were reliving the shock over again and then we had to comfort the person we called. So we asked our daughter to call and tell a short list of family and friends about the diagnosis. We probably would have told more people but we didn't have much to say besides "We have bad news."

Don, 68—transit worker

I spent a few hours with my rabbi. My faith has always been an important part of my life and it—and the community—provided me great comfort during this time.

Robert, 64—professor

Ice cream. I never eat ice cream. But if I was going to die soon, I was going to eat what I wanted. And what I wanted when I got home from the doctor's office that day was chocolate ice cream. So I ate a lot of it. Didn't make the problem go away, though.

Irene, 23—student

Common Reactions

Many people I interviewed described their thoughts dwelling on one or more of these concerns during the first days after learning their diagnosis.

PAY ATTENTION TO THAT STRONG SENSE OF URGENCY
There is one critically important characteristic of the first days after you receive a devastating diagnosis: your sense of urgency, your desire to decide on your course of action as soon as you can. You are by no means alone in having this feeling. "This was a period when my brain turned off and my emotions took over," said Elaine, a writer. "It was very dangerous. I can tell you that I did things that were entirely stupid."

Before you learned of your diagnosis, your life was fairly predictable and you felt like you had choices: to take a nap or not; to vacation with the family this spring or not; to pursue this new job or not; to visit friends on Saturday or not.

But now, nothing is predictable. You don't know what you will need to do over the next days and weeks: you may need to get tests, go to a hastily scheduled doctor's appointment, have an operation, or start a debilitating drug regimen. You don't know how any of these things will affect your ability to live your life as you planned: How much of my normal activities will I be able to do and for how long? Will I still be able to work? To go bowling? To read? To walk the dog? To pick up my grandchild?

And you don't even know when you are going to know these answers.

I hated this lack of control and predictability. So did everyone I talked to. With a few exceptions, we all felt driven to find answers quickly. And as a result, a good number of us made hasty decisions about our care that we regretted later.

Elaine recounted this story:

> My doctor was on vacation when I was diagnosed with breast cancer and I wanted to take care of it immediately, so I didn't contact him or wait the week until he returned. I went to his partner, who recommended a surgeon, who scheduled surgery immediately. But she realized during surgery that the original pathology report was wrong. And then I had difficulty healing. So it took a long time to get started on the right treatment.
>
> When he returned to this mess, my doctor asked me, "What could you have been thinking?" I think my answer then was that I thought it was straightforward and not very serious and anyone could treat this nasty little problem. But in hindsight, I think I *wanted* it to be an insignificant, solvable problem that I could snap my fingers at and it would disappear fast, since the alternative was terrifying.

My own response has generally been more garden-variety: twice I have resisted getting additional opinions about two cancers because, I told myself, seeing another doctor would delay the certain (but in hindsight, not the best) course proposed by my first doctors. I just wanted to get the operations over with and get started on whatever else I needed to do next. I didn't want to know more or hear different professional opinions. I just wanted certainty and was willing to pay a high price for it.

Ellen Stovall, president of the National Coalition of Cancer Survivorship and twice diagnosed with cancer, said that one of the most important pieces of advice her organization gives patients is to *slow down*. "It is a rare exception that any condition must be responded to within forty-eight hours. If it is so urgent, you are probably already in the hospital. For most people, it has taken years for the disease to develop to this point. Taking an extra week to see another doctor, get another opinion, and do a little more research can make all the difference between getting the wrong treatment or less good treatment, rather than the right treatment for you."

So by all means, pay attention to that sense of urgency. But also weigh the benefits of moving ahead immediately at the expense of finding the right solution, the right doctor, and the right treatment.

RECURRING THEMES

In speaking to recently diagnosed people about their responses during this period, they generally talked about how upset they were but most didn't remember much about what they did during that time. They did, however, report thinking the same thoughts over and over. Repetitive and intrusive thoughts are characteristic responses to psychological shock, so this wasn't surprising. What was interesting was that so many people reported having *similar* thoughts:

"I will always feel like this."

I couldn't imagine feeling less distressed than this. What was going to happen next was going to be terrible and painful and would mean that everything I know and love would be lost. Nothing was going to change that fact and I couldn't think beyond it.

Jacob, 41—lawyer

It is understandable that, during the hours after hearing your diagnosis, you can't imagine that this feeling of disorientation and despair could ever end. You don't know what it means for you, how you will cope, and whether you will survive.

If your imagination is anything like mine, it will rush to fill in all those blanks by finding the worst–case scenarios and dwelling on them, revisiting them over and over until they seem like reality.

I was talking with a friend whose husband had just been diagnosed with an aggressive leukemia. She told me that she felt her life is over. She knows intellectually all the statistics about how long he is likely to live and that she needs to adjust to making this time wonderful. But, she says, all this rational thought can't touch her feelings of hopelessness and her con-viction that her life has no meaning or purpose without her husband.

I encourage you to talk about feelings like these with those who love you, to seek spiritual counsel from the wise people in your life, and, if you can concentrate, read the literature of your religious or philosophical tradition. While doing so will not change the facts that face you, you may find some comfort in their perspectives.

Note that there is considerable evidence that the vast major-ity of people don't maintain the same high level of hopelessness and grief over time, and that we are remarkably resilient in the face of devastating loss and horrible events. Despite all odds, we seem to be able to move on, to take care of the things we need to, and to reconstitute our lives. This doesn't happen immediately, and most people find that they have to soldier on while in the depths of despair, acting as if they are okay. But over time, we seem to be able to adjust to many parts of this new reality.

On a more practical level, it may help to remember that many of the unknowns will start to be filled in over the next few days as you gather information and make plans to accommodate this unwelcome new condition in your life.

Marilyn, sixty–seven, a retired high school English teacher with two bouts of breast cancer behind her, had just received a diagnosis of Parkinson's disease:

> You just have to sit tight through those first forty-eight hours while your mind is racing and your spirits are in your shoes. When I got my Parkin-son's diagnosis, I used everything I knew just to keep me going: I prayed. I wrote down what I feared most. I talked to my husband and children. I walked around the block about twelve times. I knew, after all

these years of getting bad health news, that I just had to wait it out and my plan would begin to emerge—I would get a little more information and slowly, the overwhelming sadness would ebb a little and I would be able to go on.

"My behavior caused this to happen."

Many people spend hours going over their past behavior to establish the cause of their condition. They are often joined by family members and friends in their attempts to come up with an explanation for the sudden appearance of this disease. "I *know* I should have gotten that colonoscopy!" "I'm sure I got this disease because I have been so depressed and angry for so long." "I smoked for thirty years." "She just put herself under so much pressure—no wonder this happened!" "I ate too much meat and not enough vegetables." "He never took good care of himself."

Such speculation about the cause of a disease has roots in the very human need to see the world as a place that is governed by rational laws. If you can identify something you did to cause your condition, it affirms that this situation is predictable and, by extension, that the world is predictable—as opposed to random, as it feels right now. Others, by identifying behavioral causes, can convince themselves that they can avoid your fate.

As all-consuming as this line of thinking might be for you right now, try to remember two important points. The first is that diseases are caused by the convergence of many factors: your genetic makeup, your health history, your age and sex, your exposure to germs, viruses, and environmental toxins, in addition to whether you have smoked or eaten too much candy, for example. It is unlikely that your behavior is solely responsible for your disease.

The second is that the most important matter for you now is not how you may have contributed to your condition but, rather, what you do now that you know about it. Your past behavior may have influenced your health, but that is irrelevant to the challenge before you: how can you make decisions about health care and your daily responsibilities to contain or minimize the impact of this disease on your life?

"There is only one right way to respond to this diagnosis."

I hated those first few days after my diagnosis. I am the strong one in the family. I am the provider, the one who knows the answers. But there I was, the one who proved ultimately to be weak. I had no answers, only questions. I was ashamed of myself, worried about the impact of my illness on my family, and guilty about my failure as a father and as a husband.

Joaquin, 70—foundation executive

There is no right or wrong way to respond to a devastating diagnosis. We each do the best we can to take in this life-altering information.

For years, the American imagination was captured by the notion that there are predictable stages in the process of coming to terms with one's death, as proposed by Elisabeth Kübler-Ross. These stages have become part of the common vernacular and, for a time, insensitive health professionals would dismiss the anguish of their patients by labeling the stage of their behavior: "Oh, she's bargaining now."

On subsequent reflection, many observers have concluded that this mechanistic scheme isn't necessarily applicable or helpful. It is enough to know that many different emotions may swirl through you during this time, some of which may be familiar and some foreign to you. While there is a pattern of responses, each of us brings our personal experiences to this situation as each of us face our unique circumstance.

"Expressing my feelings means I have given in to the disease—and my emotions may make me worse."

We don't cry in our family, so I didn't cry and none of my kids or my wife cried. I look back and think, "What would have been so bad about crying, really?" Crying alone is so lonely. I don't think I would have been able to stop if I started. But if you can't cry with the people you love, who can you cry with?

Andrew, 57—manager

People usually express their emotions guided by what is normal in their family and in their culture. The meaning of tears, a voice raised in anger, the words "I love you" carry very different meanings depending on their social context.

This is not a normal time, however, and while controlling your emotions may help you take in the meaning of your diagnosis at your own speed, it doesn't change the fact of your condition. Expressing fear, sadness, anger, or guilt will not make your disease worse. Conversely, remaining chipper and upbeat all the time won't make it any better.

There is an intuitive—but false—link between optimism and health. The media love a tragically ill person with a stiff upper lip and plucky approach to pain. Check out the supermarket tabloids and the evening news, if you need proof. There is also a pervasive folk belief that optimism can counteract disease progression. When these links have been examined scientifically, however, they mostly evaporate.

The point is that what you are experiencing *is* awful and it *is* sad. If you express it, it may be hard for those who love you. But not doing so may isolate you at a time when you need each other's support and love the most. "Crying, raging, shouting, and talking about how you feel about this diagnosis will not hurt you physically," said David Speigel, a psychiatrist who specializes in working with women with breast cancer. "It may provide you a sense of relief and bring you closer to those you love—and may do the same for those who love you."

"Of course I'm depressed—I just got terrible news about my future!"

There is a difference between feeling sad and grieving about the loss of your future plans and feeling depressed. If you have ever been clinically depressed, you know this. If you have not, you may confuse one with the other. You may not want to get out of bed in the morning. You may have bad dreams. You may feel tearful and not care about things that yesterday meant the world to you. These are common responses to life-altering bad news.

If, however, you find your thinking shifting *from* "this is a bad situation, I have lost so much, I am so sad for myself and my family" *to* "I am a bad person; I have sinned. I deserve this disease—and I don't deserve to live," then you should seek help from a physician or mental health professional immediately.

How can you find help? One option is to call a health professional who knows you. This may be your family doctor, nurse practitioner, internist, osteopath, or other primary care clinician. Describe how you are feeling. If she feels she is capable of treating you and you know and trust her, this is the right place to start.

An alternative is to call—or ask a friend or family member to call—your local hospital and ask for names of consultation-liaison (C–L) psychiatrists. C–L psychiatrists specialize in treating the emotional and cognitive problems in people who are physically ill. This means that they are well trained in helping people manage bad medical news and understand the complexities of the interactions of an antidepressant, for example, with other drugs that a person takes or may start taking. And they understand the difference between the symptoms of a newly diagnosed disease and the responses a person is experiencing.

Yet another option: if you have seen a therapist in the past with whom you are comfortable, call him or her.

If a loved one feels hopeless and has mentioned—or you think he may be considering—hurting himself, skip these options and seek the advice of a psychiatrist. "Bring your loved one (ideally) to the private office of a psychiatrist," said Ken Gorfinkle, a psychologist who works with medically ill people. "Do your best to avoid the hospital emergency room. And as a last resort, bring your loved one to an emergency room, and do not leave him there alone."

(See appendix F for a fuller description of the range of mental health professionals who have experience in treating people facing a medical crisis.)

"Why me? This isn't fair! What did I do to deserve this?"

Western notions of fair play and justice mean that these questions are not only common but are a sign that one is feeling that the cardinal rules we assume are operating in the world have been violated. I am talking here about those deeply American assumptions about being rewarded for living a righteous life—good things happening to good people and bad things happening to bad people.

These are questions that are fundamental to our beliefs about who we are in the world, the meaning of life, and the role of God, faith, and hope. Seeking answers and solace within one's own religious or cultural tradition is the course described by person after person whom I interviewed. Most clergy see responding to spiritual crises associated with illness as part of their mandate. If you are not religious, talking with a wise friend or elder in your community might be helpful.

Common Sense Help for Getting through the First 48 Hours

These recommendations summarize the advice of professionals and opinions of individuals and their loved ones who have gone through this, and the wisdom of any mother:

This is a crisis. Treat it as one.

- Don't try to go on as though nothing is happening to you.

- Don't go to work for at least forty–eight hours, and cancel your social engagements until you get your feet back under you.

- If you need family or friends to be with you now, tell them so. Conversely, if you need to be alone, tell them that.

- If you are with others and are suddenly overcome with grief or fatigue, excuse yourself, go into another room, and close the door.

- Write down things you need to remember. You may find yourself forgetting routine appointments and simple tasks.

Protect yourself.

- You owe no explanations to anyone right now. It is your choice whom to tell and what to say, especially during these first few days. You can decide how you want to handle this later.

- Talk if you want to talk; cry if you feel like it. There is no particular benefit or harm in either.

- You are not responsible for taking care of others who are distraught at your news. Ask a family member or friend to call people you want to know about your diagnosis if you want them to know but don't want to talk right now.

- Stop searching for information online if it is confusing or frightening. You will have time to learn more later.

Don't rush to resolve your treatment plan.

- The only task you must accomplish during the first forty-eight hours is to make sure you have set up the next doctor's appointment. You need to know when you will have more information upon which to base your next steps.

- Write down questions for your doctor, employer, and insurance company as you think of them, including ones that capture your concerns about the worst-case scenarios you are imagining.

Eat.

- Even if you aren't hungry: you don't need a hunger headache.

- Drink, too. Water, for sure. Coffee or tea? Whatever you are used to. A little Scotch? Sure (but not the whole bottle).

Rest.

- Emotional stress is exhausting. If you can nap, do it. If not, lie down for a while. If you are too agitated, get up and walk around the block. If nothing else, it'll remind you that the world is just carrying on in spite of your news.

- If you can't sleep at night, do whatever you usually do to get to sleep: take a bath, warm milk, exercise, a sleeping pill. If these strategies are not successful, talk to your doctor.

Breathe.

- Take a couple of deep breaths when you remember to. Pull your shoulders down from around your ears.

Move around.

- If you usually exercise, keep it up if you feel like it. If you don't, but you feel closed in or agitated, go for a walk.

Remember: You will not always feel like this.

CHAPTER 2

Get Acquainted with Your Disease and Its Treatments

You need to know enough about your disease so that you can ask good questions and make decisions that are right for you—and so that your doctor's treatment recommendations make sense.

On the day of my diagnosis I remember being handed a printout from the National Organization of Rare Diseases. It listed everything that could happen. The nurse tried to talk us through it but we couldn't absorb anything. We took the printout home to look at it and it scared us horribly. But eventually we had to find out about what this diagnosis meant. I would sit and look at the Web sites with tears streaming down my face, sick to my stomach. I have to look at this. No one is going to do it for me.

Jean, 36—schoolteacher

THERE IS PROBABLY NO POINT in your life when it is more important to make judicious use of good scientific information—or when you feel less able to actually do that.

It humbles me to listen to people whose lives depend on finding and using good information describe how they approach this task—whether they are talking about identifying the right doctor, determining whether they are getting competent care, or choosing among treatment options. I know that it requires immense effort, energy, and resourcefulness to do this when you have received shocking news, when your life—and the lives of those you love—are irrevocably changed by a serious diagnosis of ALS or MS or cancer or stroke.

This chapter is designed to help you use your limited energy wisely to gather the information you will need over the next few weeks. It begins by laying out the reasons that you (and perhaps your family or close friends) really do need to learn the basics about your condition, its probable course, and what can be done to manage its progression. It describes how different styles of using information may influence the strategy you use to learn about your condition and its treatment.

You will find a list of questions you need to have answered in order to have a good conversation with your doctor and make good decisions, whether you plan to approach your care on a minimal need-to-know basis or you prefer to know a great deal about every aspect of your disease and treatment options. You also will find out why you want to look for good scientific information and how science makes its way to the public, as well as considerations about using what you find out.

Because people's preferences for information vary so widely and because their skills in finding and understanding complex medical information is not all the same, appendix A, "Digging Deeper: A Guide to Developing Greater Expertise," provides two strategies for finding out about your disease and possible treatments. One is for people who want to know only the basics, the other for those who want comprehensive knowledge. The appendix includes information about how to assess the quality of information, guidance about when and how to find medical articles, and Web sites and print materials that can help you make sense of them.

Why Do You Need to Know Basic Facts about Your Condition and Its Treatment?

There is a lot of new scientific information coming out but few incentives to change treatments even then. What is clear to me is that the medical industry is in some ways like any service industry. You have to show yourself as knowledgeable if you are going to get the best service—like at a garage or hotel or restaurant.

Manuel, 62—real estate investor

When you seek treatment from a physician, you are seeking to learn about—or to clarify your understanding—of your disease, its implications for your life and functioning and what treatments are available to cure it or control its progress. And you likely will want the physician to recommend a course of action that will lead to what you consider to be the best possible outcome.

You can say no or yes to a physician's recommendations. But you need some basic knowledge to be able to do so. Over the course of the next days and weeks, you will be making decisions about your treatment that will powerfully affect your future.

Right now, you may feel like you would like your partner or your spouse or parent or adult child to make all these decisions for you.

But this is *your* life. You are the one who is going to have to live every day with the consequences of an operation that may leave you incontinent or unable to drive, a treatment that may cause you to suffer but will not extend your life, or one that will provide you short-term but not long-term relief from pain.

No one but you really knows what you want or what you value most. Often there is no objectively correct answer, and you find yourself in the position of having to think about the benefits and risks of different treatments in terms of your personal preferences. So you need to have enough information to weigh the choices your doctor may offer and make decisions that are right for you.

Note that when you seek treatment from physicians who practice Western medicine, you need to know that they view the problem and its solutions within a tradition of scientific evidence and clinical experience. You may come from a culture whose concepts of health and illness are very different. You may be interested in "alternative" approaches to disease causation and treatment. But if you plan to consult with doctors who practice Western medicine, you should expect that they will view your disease and its possible treatments from this perspective.

The second reason you need to know about your condition is that, without a mental model of what is going on in your body, it is difficult to make sense of the actions you must take to participate in your treatment. If you understand generally what the pills do to keep your condition in check, you will be more likely to take them as directed and sometimes know whether they are working. If you know what a certain test will tell the doctor, you'll be more likely to show up for it or to ask about the need for it.

The third reason you need to know about your condition is that even though the United States is the world's leader in medicine, there is considerable evidence that about half of medical care delivered here is not based on what we know works best to treat and cure disease. Frequently cited studies conducted by RAND and published in the *New England Journal of Medicine* have documented this lag between medical knowledge and medical practice. Furthermore, researchers at Dartmouth Medical School have repeatedly shown that what doctors consider state-of-the-science treatment in Connecticut may be very different from what doctors do in Massachusetts or California.

"For a couple years after testicular cancer was curable, we were still seeing people dying from it in some parts of the country because their doctors didn't know there was a cure available," said Karen Antman, an oncologist and dean of the Boston University Medical School.

This does not mean that you are going to need to acquire a complete medical education to get good treatment. But it does mean that you need to know enough to ask your doctors questions about the standard treatments for your disease and to understand the answers so that you know what your choices are and can make informed decisions about them.

The fourth reason you need to know about your condition and its care is that you—and probably your partner or family members—will need to keep a vigilant eye on your care to prevent medical errors. In the United States, unlike in the United Kingdom or Canada, for example, health care is delivered through a variety of freestanding organizations and individuals: doctors in their practices, hospitals, clinics, and diagnostic centers. Currently, most patients do not have access to an electronic record that includes their entire health history, test results, and treatment plan, and which is available to any physician and hospital they designate. Each new doctor and institution you visit may have to piece together the information that is relevant to your care. It is common knowledge that such disorganization can lead to medical errors that can harm patients.

This means that you will need to know enough about your condition and your care to provide an extra pair of eyes and ears to make sure the drugs you receive are the ones that were prescribed and in the right dose, that you have told your doctor about any allergies you know about, and that the test results are in your record and have been seen by your doctors. Knowing the basics about your disease will help you keep track of what is important.

I learned from my experience that well-intentioned doctors make errors.

Andrea, 57—broadcast journalist

This probably seems like a huge responsibility, especially right now. Educating yourself about your disease can be difficult when what you really want to do is delegate the responsibility for making decisions to your doctor, for example. Furthermore, the diagnostic process sometimes moves too fast for deliberative information–gathering. "If you are going to the emergency room and then straight into surgery, there is not a lot of time to learn what this means and to discuss it," noted Janet Baradell, a psychiatric clinical nurse specialist in private practice in North Carolina.

Don't let this be an all–or–nothing proposition. You can learn the basic facts about your condition and be able to hold your own now—today—and then learn more as you need to in the next couple weeks. Or a family member or friend can pull together information for you to look over as you convalesce. Even in the midst of an acute medical crisis most people are able to acquire a workable understanding about their condition and its treatment.

Shelley McKaye, a nurse leader in pediatrics at Memorial Sloan–Kettering Cancer Center in New York City, said, "I always marvel at the ability of families, regardless of their educational level or medical sophistication, to learn this new language of medicine that they don't want to know. They learn it because they have no control and this is one way to regain a little control."

How Much Information Do You Need?

We were dealing only with what we could deal with right then. We could only deal with the diagnosis at that point: is it or isn't it? After we got the diagnosis, then we were focused only on the staging of the cancer and choosing a surgeon so we could find out how far it had spread. We didn't start thinking about treatment until we knew how bad it was.

Carmen, 37—nurse

There is evidence that we have inherent preferences for how much information we want to know about our health. Suzanne Miller, a psychologist and researcher at the Fox Chase Cancer Center, in Philadelphia, found that people tend toward being either *blunters*—those who have little interest in seeking out information or learning about their risks—or *monitors*—those who energetically track down the details about the molecular structure of their pancreas, for example.

She has found that both of these are fairly stable styles of coping. "It is as though blunters are wearing dark glasses while monitors are using a magnifying glass as they selectively attend to the world around them."

Blunters attempt to keep anxiety at bay by not attending to details that might be frightening. For example, David, a classic blunter, told me:

> I would be insulted if some yobbo read fifteen papers on theoretical physics, my own field, and then came in and asked me to help him design an experiment. And I expect the same of my doctor. I pay her. Let her sit down and tell me exactly what I need to know—what are my choices and what do they mean? That's her job. I have other things to do.

Melinda, a health policy analyst and also a blunter, said,

> I am not an information-seeker. I don't want to see pathology slides. Don't talk to me about my prognosis and don't send me articles. I don't want to be woken up at night by something that really may not apply to me. I don't want to waste my energy in fear. My job is to be calm. I pray a lot—for the right thing to happen and for the strength to deal with it, whatever it is.

Monitors are uncomfortable with the unknown. They tend to gain confidence as they gain understanding. But the monitoring style tends to rouse anxiety. People who want a lot of information sometimes have trouble figuring out when they have enough of it: they may become overwhelmed, feeling they have to absorb and factor it all into to their decisions.

For example, as Georgia, a nonprofit business executive, recalled,

I had been completely absorbed in my office since getting my diagnosis on the phone—on the Web researching things. There were literally millions of Web sites to go through! I had so many questions! I was definitely overinformed. My doctor's first advice was, "Get off the Internet! You know plenty now." It was comforting to learn that there was a fine line between information that was helpful and stuff that was just scaring me.

Under stress, people report becoming more extreme and more set in their preference for learning about their condition. If you are a blunter, you may actively resist learning more. If you are a monitor, you may spin out on the glut of information available to you, desperate that you are missing that single last piece of information that will make the difference between life and death, unable to stop searching, unable to make a decision. Over time, most monitors figure out how they can avoid this by reducing new information to a more manageable amount.

There are many stories where couples and families have different information preferences and it works out: someone will do the research and the other will participate as necessary—teenagers perform Internet searches for grandparents, a distant cousin who is a nurse tracks down references for doctors.

But I also heard heartbreaking stories where the difference in style of seeking and using information was the straw that broke the camel's back—the young woman dying of liver cancer who was estranged from her husband because he wanted to examine and expound on every journal article, every blood count, while she wanted to spend her energy enjoying the limited life she had left. Or the elderly couple responding to the husband's stroke that became divided by his faith in doctors and science, and hers in God.

It was helpful for me to do research on treatments and side effects but I didn't want to understand about my own cancer; it was too distressing and scary. I didn't want to know the survival statistics or how fast the tumors grow. I had broken up with a boyfriend just before my diagnosis. In trying to be helpful, he came over with a book that was full of this kind of information. I told him, "No, I don't want to read this." He told me he thought it was something I needed to do. And I felt like I wasn't being a good patient.

Nell, 33—lawyer

You probably have a pretty good sense of your own preference for lots or little information, as well as the preferences of those closest to you. Right now, the most important thing is for *someone* to gather the basic information, whether it is the person who was diagnosed, a family member, or a friend. *Somebody* must have it.

> My brother-in-law, who had no kids and time on his hands, did all the research and kind of spoon-fed it to me. Sometimes I could take it in and sometimes not.
>
> Harper, 42—teacher

Taking the Basic Approach

> It was amazing: one surprise after another. Nothing turned out like it was supposed to after I was diagnosed. It was always more complicated or easier or rescheduled—always different than I expected or had been told. I exercised my flexibility muscles like you wouldn't believe.
>
> Clara, 60—administrator

Hers is a common experience. Regardless of whether you are a blunter or a monitor, you need to obtain the answers to the following questions to reduce the surprise factor and put to rest at least some of the uncertainty you probably feel. Anything beyond these questions will need to be tailored by your doctor to your personal medical history, the stage of your disease, and its particular characteristics.

Fill in the answers to these questions yourself or ask a friend or family member to help you find them. Appendix A provides you with suggestions about where to find the answers, whether you are using a computer, the telephone, the library, or a bookstore.

The last time I received a serious diagnosis, I delegated this task to my husband. He was antsy to do something, and I had no patience for wading through irrelevant information to find something worthwhile. I should also admit that I wasn't that interested in hearing about what he found out. But the thing that was most helpful was that I finally convinced myself that I should say out loud to him the things that I was most scared about. Most of the time, he responded with, "Well, from what I read, I don't think that's what is going to happen. Or "I don't think we know enough about how bad this is to draw any conclusions like that. You need more tests before we'll know."

Here are the basic questions you need answers to:

- What is the name of the condition?

- What does this mean? How does this disease or condition affect the body?

- What causes this condition?

- What causes this condition to progress or get worse?

- What is the typical time course for its progression?

- What tests and procedures are commonly used to determine the course of treatment?

- What treatments are available for this condition?

- What effect does each treatment have, generally? Does it cure this condition? How often? Does it slow down its progression? How much?

- What complications and side effects are common—and uncommon—with each treatment?

You don't have to read the medical literature to answer these questions. You can ask your doctor. The explanation you will find under the disease name on the Internet using MedlinePlus, WebMD, or NIH.gov, your health plan's Web site, or the pamphlets you may request from a national nonprofit concerned with your disease should provide many answers in layman's terms. Appendix A provides you with a few more choices about where to find the basic information as well as some ideas about where to get help if you have trouble understanding it. Appendix G includes contact information for the major disease–specific nonprofit organizations.

Once you know the answers to each of these questions, you will be ready to have a discussion with your doctor about how this condition is affecting you specifically—how advanced it is; the best ways of treating it, given your age and sex and medical history; and what this means about your next steps together. On the theory of "don't jump off the bridge until you come to it," you need answers to the basic questions before you start to search for information about your own *management* of this disease; that is, how others live and cope with this condition and its treatments.

Josh Seidman, executive director of the Center for Information Therapy, said, "There is evidence that people really prefer to get their information from their physician. And people are well within their rights to ask their physician, 'Can you give me a summary of what we talked about? I'm not sure that I'll be able to remember all of it when I get home'; or 'Can you tell me where I can get more information on this that I can go over with my family?'"

Taking the Comprehensive Approach

Remember as you go forward with your search: This is a time of extreme stress. "It is not realistic to think you can compress medical school into a few weeks," noted Jeremy Boal, a geriatrician on the faculty at the Mount Sinai School of Medicine, in New York City.

If you really want to get a handle on what is going on, you should also be looking to answer the next set of questions. Answering them in detail will help you ask more sophisticated questions when you talk to your doctor.

You will want to ask:

- What are the specifics of *my* disease? (Exactly what kind of multiple sclerosis do I have? Where is the damage to my heart located? What kind of pancreatic cancer is it?)

- At what stage is my disease? (How advanced is it?)

- How does my unique medical history affect the progress and treatment of this condition? (Is my diabetes relevant? Does my family history of prostate cancer make a difference?)

- Is there anything new or emerging in the field that is promising and that I should look into now?

This information, in turn, will affect your treatment choices. The more you know about these specifics, the more efficient your search for new information will be.

People who prefer the comprehensive approach, their partners, and some health professionals who treat people like this every day, described some important considerations:

- While you can definitely improve the likelihood of getting the most effective treatment for your condition by thoroughly researching your options, *you cannot reduce the uncertainty of your situation to zero*, no matter how many articles you read, no matter how sophisticated your knowledge. Nor can your physician. Medicine—and medical science—is based on risk and probability, not certainty.

- Unless you have an acute emergency, *you have some time to collect the information you need and to digest the knowledge that will help you make better decisions*. Most people who took this approach started out slowly and built momentum as the shock of their diagnosis wore off, as they learned more about the stage and type of disease, made their treatment decisions, and approached the time to begin treatment. Sometimes this took place over two weeks, sometimes over a couple months, depending on people's readiness to absorb new information and the evolving requirements of their condition.

- That said, check every once in a while to *make sure you aren't using your information search to avoid taking important next steps*, such as scheduling an operation or deciding on a treatment. If this information-gathering phase has lasted more than six weeks or so, get help in making a decision. Your regular primary care provider may be able to help you with this, as could a wise and knowledgeable friend.

- *You are always going to have less than the optimal amount of information to make a decision.* Sometimes it is impossible to know how you will respond to a treatment until you have tried it. Your disease may change, requiring a different treatment. Some treatments take a while before it is clear whether they are effective. And a particular treatment may be too new for there to be a lot of information about it to guide your decision.

Judging the Information behind the Answers

Most information is not organized to show whether the gaps in it are because you just don't have access to that specific information or because that information doesn't exist.
—Dr. Carolyn Clancy, Director, U.S. Agency for Healthcare
Research and Quality

In the United States, we are both blessed and cursed with a flood of health information. Blessed because there is so much available and cursed because even if you know a lot about science and health, it is hard to know whether what you have found is good information.

The rest of this chapter and appendix A provide guidance about finding and judging the quality of information about medical conditions and their treatments. It does not include information that addresses the quality or effectiveness of programs that provide support in coping with serious diagnosis. These topics are discussed in chapters 9 and 10.

*How can I best learn what research says about
my disease and its treatment?*

Often, research is published as articles in medical and scientific journals. These journals remain one of the main ways doctors communicate with one another about advances in medicine. Medical journals can be a valuable source of information for those who want as full an understanding as possible of their condition. But there are a few things you should know about medical journals:

- They are not all created equal. The big-name journals like the *New England Journal of Medicine* and the *Journal of the American Medical Association* publish only high-quality studies relevant to the current practice of medicine, and that have been carefully reviewed and evaluated by researchers and physicians. But there are 4,844 medical journals in the National Library of Medicine's online database, Medline, some of which contain high-quality research pertaining to a specific disease and others that contain lesser-quality research. It is difficult to assess the quality of journals, and the results of the most reliable efforts to do so are available only for a fee. If you are going to be reading original research articles, check out the journal's policy on accepting papers. This will give you a sense of whether the journal publishes research that has been reviewed by other experts in the field—in other words, "peer-reviewed" research. If you are unfamiliar with a publication and have found a promising article in it, you may wish to inquire about a journal's "impact factor," usually available through university and hospital libraries or through the company ISI. This number will give you an idea of how a journal stacks up relative to the top-ranked ones.

- It takes skill to make sense of what you read in a medical journal. Unless you are medically trained—and often even if you are—findings that are published in medical journals are difficult to penetrate. The writing is technical, the pages are full of statistical analyses, and what you read is probably only one piece of the very large puzzle that is your disease. You can, however, gain the skills to read reports of scientific studies that will make them more valuable to your understanding, although it is not realistic to believe you will become expert at this in a few weeks. Appendix A provides sources you can use to become a better reader. If nothing else, you can gain a basic understanding of how medical studies explain the risk involved in certain treatments, the meaning of relative and absolute risk, and how to recognize the best-designed scientific studies. But if this task still seems overwhelming, drop it. You may just find it easier and less stressful to put your energies into choosing a doctor and a health-care team that you trust to gather and interpret these studies for you.

- It is difficult to draw conclusions about what specific study findings mean for *you*. A study might include a group of people who are similar to you in one way but different from you in very important ways. This makes it difficult to personalize the findings of any study to your

unique situation. Even well-designed clinical trials sometimes produce findings that conflict with one another and
you may want to look for systematic reviews or meta-
analyses that summarize the effects of a treatment across
many studies.

Physicians get much of their scientific information from medical journals.
Most doctors read some medical journals that describe the latest
research about the cause, diagnosis, and treatment of diseases. In
addition, physicians' knowledge comes from book and laboratory
learning in medical school, their training (treating patients while
being supervised), their overall experience treating patients over
the years, and their continuing education, which is required for
all United States physicians (except in the District of Columbia).
When your doctor is talking to you, all this—plus his knowledge
about you, your medical history, and your disease—informs what
he is saying.

Note, however, that doctors vary in their experience in treating life-altering conditions; a specialist may *only* treat patients
with variations of your condition, while a general internist may
only treat one or two patients with it in the course of a year.
Some physicians are more curious than are others; some are
more careful about staying on top of new treatment developments than are others. Furthermore, a family practitioner or internist may not feel comfortable describing all the treatment
options available for prostate cancer or lupus, for example. Most
people who have a life-altering condition consult at least one
doctor who is a specialist whose expertise is in one kind of disease. (See chapter 4 to find out more about this.)

*Government, health plans, and nonprofit disease groups and commercial in-
terests "package" the results of research studies.* There is broad recognition
that most of us don't know as much as our doctors do. Yet at the
same time that there is increasing public interest in having accurate knowledge about health and health care, we ironically, have
less access to physicians who can help us sort through our treatment options. Further, there is growing evidence that patients
who participate in decisions about their health care do better.

As a result, considerable investments have been made recently to make solid scientific information available to us in a format we can understand and put to use. The federal government,

the health voluntaries like the American Heart Association and the Project Inform national hotline for people with HIV/AIDS, as well as health plans like Aetna, United HealthCare, and Kaiser Permanente, have gone into the patient information business in a big way. Between these various sources, it is likely that you have easy access not only to good basic information about your condition but may also be able to talk on the telephone to a trained advice nurse or counselor who can help you find material and can answer initial questions. (See appendix G for more information on the specific services each source can offer and which formats—mailed pamphlets, online libraries, and local referrals—are available.)

A particularly valuable overlooked resource is the short summaries by experts that review the most recent studies relating to a particular condition and its treatment and who exactly might benefit from the treatment. These summaries often deal with a very narrow and specific question (the benefits of angioplasty for blocked vertebral arteries, for example) and are often aimed directly at physicians to help make decisions in treating their patients based on the latest evidence.

The government's National Cancer Institute includes such summaries on its Web site as "PDQs" (Physician Data Queries), and insurance companies like Aetna produce guideline summaries under the name Clinical Policy Bulletins. Check your own health plan's Web site or call the advice line if you are curious. You can find more information on them in appendix A.

The media report on new scientific findings. TV, radio, newspapers, and Web sites are full of news reports of new advances in health. This week alone, I saw six news reports about progress in finding new treatments for serious diseases.

If you watch these carefully over time, you will observe a couple of important things:

- First, contradictory findings are frequently reported. How much exercise *do* you have to do to reduce your risk of heart disease? Last week it was thirty minutes of intensive activity, this week it's fidgeting all the time. Which diet works better—low fat or low carb? Is coffee a lethal substance or a healthy food? The answers to any of these questions will depend on what week you ask them, because they change depending on the results of the most recent study.

And therein lies one caution about the news media as a source of information about your condition: News reports are often about findings from single new studies. If you are a scientist working on heart disease, for example, new findings about the effect of exercise are one more tiny piece in the large complex mosaic of your knowledge. They will add incrementally to what you know. If you are not a scientist—if you are a journalist or a member of the public—you often lack the context into which this new single study fits. There may have been many other studies that came to a different conclusion; this study may be smaller or larger, whatever. The point is that news articles report on developments you may want to ask your doctor about, but rarely do they tell the whole story.

- Second, the news media have an optimistic bias in reporting on health news. How often have you read a headline about a new cure for some serious disease? Contrast this with news of findings that long-standing treatments don't make a difference. While recent news about the ineffectiveness of some familiar drugs has made a small dent in this optimism, such news has only recently made its way from the business pages to the front page of the newspaper.

Scientists, doctors, and patients write books to describe current scientific understanding of diseases and treatments. The health section of your local bookstore, library, or online book merchant will include books that may be relevant to your quest to understand your condition. Resource books like *Dr. Susan Love's Breast Book* (Perseus, 2000) and *Dr. Patrick Walsh's Guide to Surviving Prostate Cancer* (Warner, 2001) focus on presenting scientific information clearly in a way that can help you make decisions. Self-help books usually provide an accurate scientific picture of the disease but focus more on its management over time. Celebrity and patient accounts of their experiences with your condition rarely purport to provide scientific information.

It is important to remember that anyone can publish a book, Web site, or magazine article, and write whatever he or she wishes, be it true or false. There is no reader protection against false health information published in books, unlike information published by the government, nor is there a requirement for peer review by other scientists as there is in medical journals. In other words, authors of books are able to make claims about products and treatment approaches and their effectiveness without any proof whatsoever. So it is wise to choose with care the periodicals, books, and Internet sources you use to learn about your condition.

There are a few ways to increase the likelihood that you are reading good-quality information in books. First, look for authors who have a formal relationship with a known university or medical school. Then look at the credentials of the authors:

- Where were they educated and when?

- With what universities, medical schools, and hospitals are they currently affiliated?

- What kind of recognition and awards have they received from their peers in professional societies and universities?

- What professional experience do they cite that is relevant to the subject of the book?

Advertisements cite scientific studies to bolster claims of the effectiveness of products. Whether on TV, radio, or Web sites, the purpose of advertising is to sell a product. The pharmaceutical industry has, over the past decade, invested heavily in advertising to patients—and potential patients—with the goal of educating the public about the potential benefits of their products. Studies have shown that such advertising does not often benefit patients—that it is aimed at getting people to request a specific prescription drug when there is no evidence that it is any more effective than a generic one or one that is available over the counter and cheaper. There is some evidence, however, that it sometimes encourages people to talk to their doctor or nurse practitioner about problems they might otherwise have ignored.

In addition, manufacturers of a wide variety of health products also advertise their benefits, often without regulation. You can find a large array of medicines and devices online, especially ones that claim to be able to cure almost any serious condition imaginable. These claims are not regulated and there are no protections, so buyer beware.

A Short Note about the Internet

I'm so glad to be alive in the age of the Internet. My dad died of ALS and after his death, I found copies of all these letters he had sent to doctors all over the country asking them to explain what was happening to him. He had to wait for the *mail* to find out.

Manuel, 62—real estate investor

The Internet is a valuable tool for tracking down health information. Eight in ten Internet users surveyed by the Pew Internet and American Life Project say they have looked for health information online. Furthermore, all the different channels through which scientific research makes its way to us converge on the Internet. Online, you can find original articles, physician advice, books, information packaged for consumers, and advertisements.

"People run to the computer like it is an oracle," stated a physician/health plan executive. "But they don't have the background to separate the wheat from the chaff. What people take away is often unintelligible—it is like a talisman to them. They come in with some wild ideas about treatment." Worse, much of the health information online is inaccurate or deliberately misleading. This is a serious limitation, especially for those with limited medical knowledge.

Clearly, there is a big difference between having access to a computer and the Internet, and knowing how to search in a way that gets you accurate information quickly. It takes a good deal of skill and practice to do so generally, and, even if you are an expert at tracking down, say, the latest information about the college football draft or downloading music that you love, finding good health information may be a challenge.

That said, the Internet offers a wealth of good information and access to expertise from all over the world—not only of scientists and physicians, but also of patients and family members who have followed each development in the treatment of disease, who have experience with all the treatments, and who are willing to offer advice, support, and understanding to others with their condition. The online community of patients is as diverse as society at large; off and on, it proved to be an invaluable aid of many people I interviewed.

If you do not have easy access to a computer or feel you have neither the interest nor skills to search for information online right now, you can ask a family member or acquaintance to help you. Think about it before you delegate such research. There can be unforeseen consequences, as Eleanor, sixty-four, a consultant, found:

> I asked my teenage stepson to do some research on the Web for me. He went on all the Web sites and it scared the daylights out of him!

Sometimes librarians can help with Internet searches. Every public library in the country has Internet access. Check with your hospital to see if the medical librarian there can be of help to you. If an Internet search is not possible or desirable, your doctor, the library, national telephone lines, and the local chapter of the health voluntary organization that specializes in your disease can get you good information to get started.

If you are fairly comfortable negotiating your way around the Internet but have not spent a lot of time looking for health information, you may want to take a look in appendix A, in the section on understanding the technical language to help you streamline your search.

CHAPTER 3

Involve Others

Your aim is to involve friends and family in ways that will strengthen and sustain you and not distract you or sap your energy in the days ahead.

Speech is civilization itself—the word, even the most contradictory word, preserves contact—it is silence that isolates.
—Thomas Mann, *Magic Mountain*

D O YOU WANT TO TELL anyone else about your diagnosis? You don't have to, you know. Many people find that doing so brings much-needed help and support during these first days, whereas others find it too painful to talk about right now. Some are embarrassed or just feel like it is no one else's business. Others decide to wait until they know a little more about what they are going to do before they tell anyone.

You have a choice about this.

This chapter approaches the larger questions of involving others and of thinking ahead about your wants and needs in the coming days. It is divided into three main sections. The first explores what it means—and what it takes—to tell friends and acquaintances about your diagnosis right now. It describes how people made different decisions and why; it identifies some common responses; and it discusses the tough problem of asking for help from friends.

The second discusses some of the ins and outs of involving family—adult children, little children, adolescents, parents—in the process you are going through. Although it is often unrealistic to think you can conceal your illness from family members living with you, there are ways of approaching their involvement that you might want to consider before informing them.

The third section talks about why you might need extra help from friends and family in the days ahead, and gives you a strategy for asking for that help.

Telling Others

My own experience with this was different with each illness. The first time I was diagnosed with cancer, I was twenty years old and was so amazed by it, I think I told people just so that I could convince myself it was real, along the lines of "Can you believe what's happened to me?" I was pretty undiscriminating in who I told: gas station attendant, person in front of me in the movie line, basically, whoever came in range.

The second time, I just could not believe this had happened *again*. Denying that it had, describing it as not so serious, and dawdling about getting treatment were ways I tried to convince myself that it really hadn't. I told only a few people, and I felt ashamed of it—I was ashamed of myself and thought I had done something to cause it.

The third time I received a devastating diagnosis, I had gone to the doctor with puzzling symptoms and was hospitalized immediately. Even now I don't fully comprehend the threat to my life. I experienced it as a bad case of flu, although it was an acute heart condition. My husband did all the telling this time—he had a phone list of family and a few close friends, and would work his way through it every couple days so that the people who needed to know did.

And the fourth time—well, the fourth time was the time that made me decide to write this book. By then, I should have been an old hand at this. I was very well connected with the doctors and hospitals in my community, I knew how and where to find out what I needed to know, and I had gone through this three times before. But it turned out that all that privilege, knowledge, and experience were not that helpful as I launched into unraveling the implications of *this* diagnosis.

Here are some accounts of different ways people have handled telling others:

"I told everyone."

I have an outgoing, field marshal–type personality and despite the fact that I felt devastated, I told everyone—no secret. I didn't want this to be a dirty word, a dirty disease for others. This was the right thing for me. This is who I am. To get the love and support I needed, I had to tell people… it was a really positive thing.

Meryl, 57—college president

Look—I'm single and I have a child and I'm scared that I'm going to die. I need all the help I can get. And I have been amazed and gratified by what people are willing to do for us. Really—they have come forward with these generous offers from every nook and cranny of my life. I would never say I am glad this happened, but it really has opened my eyes to the generosity of people.

Hannah, 37—teacher

I sent out an e-mail to sixty or so friends after I realized that every time I told someone in person, I would re-experience this whole range of emotions. And then I had to watch the expression on the face of the person who was watching my own pain.

Barrie, 49—cancer researcher

"I told no one."

At the time, my husband had just taken on an important, highly visible job and we were certain that if his illness became known, his board would have lost confidence in him and he probably would been asked to step down. So except for our [adult] kids, we told no one. We found a plausible alternative diagnosis and stuck with that. Fortunately, he was able to get through the treatment with few outward signs of illness.

Ann, 59—museum curator

I found it hard to tell people. I'm somewhat of a private person. My whole firm didn't know. Even telling the few people I did was difficult—it was like scuffing scabs off a wound. It made me upset knowing how upset they would be.

Nell, 33—lawyer

For a long time I didn't want to impose on my children. They have such full lives with their jobs and their own kids. I eventually told them and they kind of moved in and started managing everything.

Ruth, 74—homemaker

"I told a few people."

The very first day I told a couple very close friends. After that, I wasn't secretive, but I didn't tell people proactively. But I'd let people know if they asked. I just didn't want to become a poster child for this condition. I didn't want everyone's first greeting to be that deep, meaningful "How ARE you?"

Elaine, 60—artist

It was no one else's business. Plus, what was I going to say—"I have cancer but I don't know what kind or how bad or what it's going to do to me or what my treatment is"? I figured I would tell the people who needed to know when I had some of the answers. Just the thought of telling my mother until after I had begun treatment was too much for me to handle. I did tell my boss once I had a sense of how the treatment was going to affect my work performance.

Don, 68—transit worker

Many people spoke of receiving profound advice and hearing expressions of love and support that were meaningful and comforting in the days that followed. Eliana Horta, a clinical nurse specialist who spent much of her career in Chile and New York City caring for people who had just received a devastating diagnosis said, "Are you prepared to tell others? If not, ask yourself what is behind this drive. Is it because you are a private person? Because you are ashamed? Guilty? Don't want people to feel sorry for you? Feel that people will ostracize you? Once you realize what is behind your concerns, it is yours to decide. Your family has nothing to say about what is the right choice."

She went on: "The most painful part of illness is the loneliness—the feeling of being so profoundly alone—seeing others' self-interest and realizing how you are connected to others but are still fundamentally alone. Think carefully before you live your life with such a secret."

IF PEOPLE KNOW, THEY ARE GOING TO RESPOND

During a health crisis, family members, friends, and even distant acquaintances often rise above the everyday fray and behave with extraordinary generosity, warmth, and compassion. Many will offer to help and will follow through. They will send notes and flowers; they will call and e-mail; they will be sensitive to the crisis or emergency and the stress it places on your family and will be creative in how they pitch in to help.

But sometimes the responses fall slightly outside of the realm of helpful. They may even be irritating or distressing. Many people I interviewed brought this up—enough of them so that it is worth discussing briefly. They usually mentioned at least a couple of the responses listed below. Two things were interesting about this: First, that so many people reported hearing these responses again and again. And second, for every person who found one of these responses offensive or irritating, there was one who found the same response immensely comforting.

I am the first to admit that my own responses to some of these comments have not always been tactful or kind. My impulse to whack the next person who tells me I'm going to be just fine has too often barely made it into the only slightly less offensive response: "How do you know, big shot?" I hope that knowing what to expect can soften the irritation and the pain inflicted thoughtlessly by others, so here are some common responses you have probably already heard:

"You must *see my doctor. He is the only/best one to treat X!" "What you want to do is start Y treatment immediately. Here is the Web site information—I promise—It'll cure you!"* Such advice is often forcefully offered but may be helpful and point you toward options you didn't know you had. After all, word of mouth is one of the main ways people

hear about doctors and treatments, whether for a serious diagnosis or a minor one. And, there are other people who have really become experts in their own cancer—who have done all the research, who know all the doctors, who have firsthand experience with care at different hospitals. This is the kind of person whom you ask about which dishwasher to buy because you trust that she has done all the research, looked at *Consumer Reports*, done quality and price comparisons, and bought, tested, and returned several models. Finding people whose judgment and experience you trust can be a great help.

But there are also a few things to keep in mind about personal referrals:

- One of the great things about modern medicine is that we know so much that many treatments are personalized to the individual, depending on the stage of one's disease, one's age and sex, medical history, and preferences. What was right for your friend may not be right for you.

- Individuals who refer you to their own doctor may be basing their recommendation only on their own experience. While it is wonderful that they have good rapport with their physician and to feel they received effective treatment, those positive feelings are only a part of the information you need about a doctor to know whether she or he is the right one for you. (See chapter 4 for the other kinds of information you might consider in choosing your physician.)

- There are many ways to respond to a bad diagnosis, and medical treatment is the most common but by no means the only way. You will get advice about diet, exercise, massage therapy, and alternative medicine of various sorts, along with accounts of their effectiveness. Again, *your* needs and preferences will determine what you do with this information. (See chapter 9 for more about alternative medicine choices.)

"My friend's aunt had exactly your condition and she's fine." (Alternatively, *"and she died after long and painful treatment."*) As you no doubt know by now, it is extraordinary how many people come out of the woodwork as having—or knowing someone who has—exactly the disease or condition that you have!

These stories come with the territory. It is hard to tell people you aren't interested in hearing them when they are recounting them with the best of intentions. If they had anything more helpful to say, they would be saying it instead. If the stories start to bother you, distract yourself by keeping count of how many times you hear the same one over the first few weeks. Seriously—who *knew* your condition was so popular!

Some people will be very upset by your news. They may carry on, weep, and expect you to cry with them or they may become distant or remote. You know how frightening this diagnosis is for you and those closest to you? Occasionally, even those who are not that close to you will experience your bad news as though it were theirs; that this is happening to someone they know means that it could happen to them and it scares them. That reaction is upsetting at a time when you are concerned about yourself and you have told others about your condition in the hope that they would recognize this is a real emergency for you.

People who respond to your news by withdrawing can be hurtful. Reaching out to those who have walked away from you during this time is tricky, and it may be that you should let it rest for a while rather than risk a rebuff. You have more urgent things to attend to. Later on, you may want to say something along the lines of "I was hurt when I knew you knew about my diagnosis but I didn't hear anything from you."

"I'm sure everything is going to be just fine." Most times, this is just a careless misphrasing of "I *hope* everything is going to be okay."

"Your disease will change your life." "This disease will show you what's really important." "This condition is really a blessing, you'll see." It is a real tribute to human resilience that people can grow and change in the face of serious illness. And it may be that knowing this can happen will be a beacon of hope for you during the days ahead, because each person who tells you this is proof that survival is possible. But some days, it may just sound weird, since you don't yet know if you are going to live to appreciate these lessons or are unsure that you will be able to adjust to the changes in your relationships and life that the disease demands.

Hearing you will see your disease as a blessing is a little like a concert pianist telling you "You'll be able to play beautiful music just like me after you practice all day every day for twenty years" when you can't read music, don't have a piano, and quite frankly, would rather be skiing.

It may be too early for you to feel like your diagnosis is a good thing quite yet, and you may never feel that way.

"Your disease is God's will or punishment." "You don't go to church enough." "You must be a bad person to deserve this fate." Being in the middle of a health crisis is difficult enough without being told that you caused it. And many people beat themselves up quite nicely trying to find a behavioral or spiritual explanation for their disease without assistance from others.

If faith is important to you and you have been wrestling with doubts like these, you may find it helpful to talk with a member of the clergy. Hospital chaplains have lots of experience talking with people about such concerns, as has your own minister, priest, rabbi, or imam, if you have one (see chapter 9). If you are not religious and have been thinking about spiritual issues, you might talk about them with someone you consider wise, whether or not he or she is associated with a religious community.

"You are so brave! I don't know how you do it! If I had to do what you are doing I'd be under the table." A number of young mothers reported hearing this repeatedly. Cindy, a thirty-six-year-old homemaker, wishes she could respond: "You know what? You don't know what I do when you leave and I'm alone sitting in my room. It is not a *brave* thing to put dinner on the table for my family or to put the laundry in the washing machine. Being sick wasn't a choice and neither is this. You just do it."

"You realize that you having this disease means that now I have to worry about getting it, too." Or *"Your illness is really inconvenient for me: it came right in the middle of my busiest season at work!"* The sudden diagnosis of a serious disease is not only reliably disruptive and inconvenient for everyone involved, but it can also be threatening to individual family members, since it may mean that their own risk for this disease is greater than they believed. Those closest to you sometimes feel the least inhibited in letting you know about the negative impact of your condition on them.

"You only have X disease? What are you so upset about? I have Y—that's much worse than what you have and I'm not upset at all." Competitive

comments are unfortunately common—one of the unexpected downsides of talking with others who have a similar condition. Such comments make me feel weak and stupid, as though I am a wimp to be so upset by my paltry little cancer! But I know from my experience and from the accounts of those I interviewed that each person's diagnosis carries its own meaning, confers its own dislocations, and causes its own pain.

Involving Families

Family constellations are unique and as part of their history each family develops ways of coping with crises.

—Don Schumacher, president, National
Hospice Foundation

This is a time when many families rally round, putting aside grudges and disagreements, and abandoning other plans so that they can show up and help out. This is, after all, quintessentially what "family" means in most cultures.

But any time you get that many people with that many, close, complicated, long-standing relationships focused on one highly emotional, highly charged problem—in this case, the condition of the person with the diagnosis—it gets tricky. Despite the uniqueness of each family situation, however, there were patterns in the way families I talked with reacted that might help you anticipate some of the responses of your own family during this time.

To begin with, styles of coping differ within families. A "coping style" refers to one's inherent tendency to act consistently in a certain way in response to stress. Since coping is what you are doing during this time, it is worthwhile to note a couple things about coping styles:

First of all, you don't have a lot of choices about your coping style. If your wife is a person who generally withdraws into herself in stressful situations, she probably isn't going to suddenly change and say, "Hey! I think I'll try out a new way of doing this—perhaps I'll experiment with an outgoing personality." You might wish that your wife had more interest in talking about what is going on and she might indeed make a good faith effort to do so. But if withdrawing is generally her style, then this is probably going to be her main response right now.

Different coping styles can also be the source of conflict within families, especially during this time of heightened emotional upset. It is easy to feel that a person could cope in a more functional way if he chose to. Your partner's style looks like denial to you—or your partner says you tend to be hysterical, or that you are a know-it-all who is trying to compete with the doctor. The result can be harsh words at exactly the wrong time.

Privacy can be another source of disagreements. When two people make a serious lifetime commitment to each other, they bring to the relationship a set of norms and expectations about privacy, including what kind of information is shared among family members.

> If I need a procedure done, I don't tell anyone. I don't tell my husband because he worries and tells his family. This humiliates me. I find it degrading and obnoxious even when something consequential has happened. His family is built in a way that these things are talked about. It is cultural, familial, and personal. And it drives me nuts.
>
> Jan, 60—physician

And then there are the talkers and nontalkers. Again, it doesn't take a health crisis to recognize that every family has somebody who grunts and somebody who launches into her life story when you ask how her day went. But this can be particularly noticeable and difficult when you want to discuss (or not discuss) one of the most serious topics of your life.

"There are real differences in families between the talkers and nontalkers. The silent ones feel talkers are torturing them while the talkers feel silent ones are not dealing with what's happening. You can't make a talker a nontalker and vice versa," said Paula Rauch, a psychiatrist who works with medically ill children and adults at the Massachusetts General Hospital in Boston.

> I longed to have a conversation with my husband: What was he thinking? Was he as scared as me? What were we going to do? But he wanted none of it. Football on TV, that was it. And silence.
>
> Christy, 50—retail clerk

It is normal that individuals respond in different ways to a crisis. There is no right way. What you have to watch out for is when one of you does things that put you at risk or hurts others. See what you can do to be kind to each other while you are all so upset.

> On day three after my diagnosis, my two kids marched into the living room and the eleven-year-old put his hands on his hips and said, "Okay, you guys want to tell us what's going on?" I told them the diagnosis, the test that I was going to have that day, and that I was going to be fine but that I had to go to the doctor, have some procedures, take some medicine.
>
> Georgia, 46—nonprofit business executive

There are never successful family secrets.

Kids always know that something is up. Even if they are too young to understand, they overhear things and pick up on the emotional tone. So if you have children who are living at home or who are in college or are otherwise dependent on you, you need to tell them something about what is happening. If they are over the age of three or four, the notion that you can't tell them is unrealistic.

"Parents know their children," notes Paula Rauch, of Massachusetts General Hospital. "This is one more transition or disruption in the kid's life. How did your child react to the first day of school? How easy is it for her to adjust to a change in plans? Use your knowledge of your children's temperament to figure out how to communicate with them about your diagnosis. You will learn as things develop."

Catherine Monk, a psychologist in the Department of Psychiatry at Columbia University, in New York City, says there are a few basic pointers about talking with children about a devastating diagnosis:

- Both parents need to be on the same page, giving the same message and same information.

- In the midst of a crisis, it is easy to become absorbed by the details and want to describe everything. It is really important to be aware of the different roles of kids and adults right now. Children shouldn't know everything you are thinking and feeling. When you tell children that a parent is sick, the story needs to explain the emotional upset but leave the kids out of the treatment decisions and physical details that may involve aspects of your body you don't ordinarily discuss in depth with them.

- Try to be open to questions and be attuned to their dreams, play, and tangential questions that don't seem at first glance to have anything to do with your diagnosis.

- You don't need to ask children directly how they are doing. Make general observations, float hypotheses: "I was thinking about what I told you about mom being sick. Lots of times when kids hear that their mother is sick at first they don't really think about it but later on—like at night—they do and they get really scared."

- It's important to hold on to rules of the family. Rules help kids feel safe. Try to maintain bedtimes, curfew, and chores. Otherwise children will feel that things are falling apart.

- When you tell your child that you or the other parent is sick, this is the *start* of a conversation that will continue over time. The meaning of your illness will change as you learn more, as you progress in your illness and treatment, and as your child develops. Think about what your kid was doing, what she was interested in, and what she was playing with eight months ago; they change so fast! What your illness means today is different from what it will mean even a few weeks from now.

- You may not feel you handled talking to your kids about your illness perfectly but you will have many opportunities over time. This is not a one-time conversation.

Involving Young Children

You are at the center of your children's world and when your strength and wisdom is threatened, it reverberates through their lives. They are terrified that they may lose you and all that you mean to them: stability, caring, and normalcy.

Telling your child you are sick is actually quite simple. Speaking honestly and using words children can understand, say "I am sick right now and we are going to the doctor to do everything we can to help me get better."

My son knew something was up. I talked to him about it once but then realized that I hadn't used the word *cancer*. So I told him again using the word. He said, "Mom—you have cancer? Don't touch me!" and ran away. So I rushed to explain cancer isn't contagious. He said "Mom, I was just playing a game!" and then we ended playing a tickly hide-and-seek cancer-monster game.

Hannah, 37—teacher

They will ask questions you can't answer, most notably, "Will you be okay? Will you get better? Will you die?" Your answer is, "I hope I will be okay and not die and I am going to do everything I can to make sure I will be fine."

But they will also ask questions you can answer. Young children want to know what is going to happen in the next twenty-four hours, not twenty-four months. They want to know if you will pick them up at school tomorrow and whether they can still be a princess for Halloween on Friday. When it comes right down to it, they really don't understand what your diagnosis means to you or to them and, as a result, their response may be disarmingly cold-blooded: "I know you have MS but I have to do my science project."

Parents sometimes try to protect their young children from the news of a bad diagnosis by not telling them that they are sick, but the parent's distress combined with his or her silence about its source scares them more. Children are frightened when they are not included in something upsetting and tend to think that it is about them, that *they* did something wrong—for example, "If only I hadn't made my mom so mad all the time—if I had gone to bed on time—she wouldn't be sick."

This is not surprising: adults frequently blame themselves and worry that they somehow caused their own disease. You may want to directly address this blame dynamic if you think it is going on. We often blame ourselves when things happen that we can't control but it's really important to remember that "you are not to blame for me being sick—and I am not to blame."

Make sure, above all, that you tell your children that you don't want to leave them. This is a time to tell your children you love them again and again.

> As I was leaving for the hospital, they cried, "Don't leave us, Mommy. Don't let them hurt you. Don't have cancer!" I could not breathe. They were so upset and I told them to pray for themselves and me. I told them that God would carry them through the night and into the day. I promised to see them in the afternoon. I promised to hold them and hug them forever. I made promises that I did not know if I could keep.
>
> Maral, 44—writer

Involving Adolescents

The need to tell your adolescent children what is going on is no less pressing than with small children. For many adolescents, who may be less interested in their family and more concerned with their friends right now, the overriding concern is conforming to their peers—except when *they* choose not to conform. Have you ever seen that bumper sticker JUST BECAUSE SOMETHING IS AN EMERGENCY FOR YOU DOESN'T MEAN IT'S AN EMERGENCY FOR ME? That just might be the sign plastered on your adolescent's forehead.

> My daughter was entering her teenage years and acted as though the world revolved around her. She insisted that my cancer was not an issue for her. A few days ago I mentioned that she had never told me how she feels about my cancer. She replied, "Your cancer doesn't affect me." She just won't talk about it. She's having a rough adolescence, though.
>
> Cindy, 36—homemaker

Outward indifference sometimes characterizes adolescents' immediate responses to an urgent health crisis in their parents or grandparents. The illness of a family member undermines their fledgling independence; fear of what might happen pulls them back into their family just at the point when they thought they were becoming adult. "This is a time when under the best of circumstances, kids need their parents to be steady so they can push them away," said Catherine Monk, of Columbia University. "So when parents are unsteady or appear weak, adolescents get mad. They feel very threatened by being drawn back into the close relationship with their parents. The anger that a parent is ill can make them feel guilty."

Jill, a minister, described how her daughter was fifteen when she had abdominal surgery.

> While I was in the hospital, she went out and got a tattoo of a butterfly on her stomach, though she denied it had anything to do with me. This started a cycle of some difficult years—she was determined to be independent and I was determined not to take any crap.

The illness of a family member also makes teenagers different from their friends. They may need to be home to care for younger siblings while you are having tests done or they may feel they must be there in case something bad happens; at the same time they may hate being torn away from the highly charged world of school and friends.

Regardless of how adolescents are negotiating this stage of their life, they will sense that something is wrong and need to know what it is, lest they believe it is about themselves and something they have done wrong. They need honest, straightforward information in the same way younger kids do. They need to know what is going to happen next and how this will affect them. They may be more interested in the details of your diagnosis and the decisions you must make than are younger children, but not necessarily.

Because they are older, they may already have ideas about what your condition means. For example, they may think that having cancer means you will die like their classmate's dad did, or that having MS means you will be in a wheelchair starting tomorrow. It is worthwhile to find out what they know about the disease in general and to give them a more realistic sense of what your diagnosis may lead to in the near future—what tests you need to have, what you think the treatment might be. Your aim is to help them not jump to conclusions but, rather, to contain their own panic and fear at the prospect of losing you.

Parents of children of all ages talked about finding a counselor for their children. Hannah, the teacher, said,

I took my son to a therapist and now that I am feeling better, he is less frightened. But I think he needs that scaffolding around him for when something happens.

"Many kids like a scheduled time to talk to a grown-up but others just want a point person," noted Paula Rauch, of Massachusetts General Hospital. "This may be a time when you are so upset that you can't talk about grieving and loss with your teenager. If you are unable to talk with him right now," she says, "You may want to make sure there is another adult around who he *can* talk to. With younger kids, you can say 'Not now,' but teenagers take that as rejection."

Involving Adult Children

In many families, adult children want and expect to be involved in any illness or crisis. They can be a tremendous help in making decisions, accompanying you to the doctor, or even running out for groceries. "If you receive a devastating diagnosis and decide to handle it yourself and don't tell your kids, you may be failing to take advantage of an important support system," said Eleanor Ginzler, director of Livable Communities at AARP.

While I was still recovering, my dad was diagnosed with prostate cancer. I flew out to go with him to his doctor. The doctor told me later that it was really important that I was with him because he was so frightened. I would never have known he was scared had the doctor not told me. My father didn't say anything about being upset.

Barrie, 49—cancer researcher

Nevertheless, the responses of adult children may be unexpected, as I heard over and over again:

Our children were shocked that one of their parents might be sick. They needed so much support! Each one responded differently and all of them grew up a lot. They all became part of the team.

Eleanor, 64—consultant

> One of my sons just took over. He managed everything. He treated me
> like I am incompetent. He alienated the other children. He was critical
> of the doctors. He thought he was doing the right thing. You know that
> road to hell...
>
> Adele, 70—retired teacher

Some people choose not to involve their adult children because they don't want to feel like a burden on their families. Eleanor Ginzler, of AARP, says this is particularly true of women over sixty. "Sometimes women don't share this information because they fear their children will be inconvenienced or because they are catapulted into action by the crisis and don't feel they have the time or emotional energy to involve their children."

And sometimes older women—and men—don't tell *or* take charge. This is a source of family conflict, says Ms. Ginzler, because "they don't tell but the kids want to know. The mother thinks she is handling it just fine the way she wants to but the kids want to help and go into hyperspace that she won't let them."

Remember: no matter what response you get from your adult children, *you* are still the one in charge of deciding how to handle your diagnosis.

Telling Your Parents about Your Diagnosis

> My first reaction to my diagnosis was that I was grateful it wasn't my
> wife or my daughter. My second one was that I was glad I didn't have to
> tell my parents.
>
> Bert, 54—endocrinologist

This sentiment was echoed again and again by people whose parents were no longer living as they imagined the blow their diagnosis would have dealt to their parents. Those with older parents still living really struggled with the question of whether and how to tell them that they were ill:

> It was hard telling my mom. She was in the early stages of Alzheimer's
> and she just couldn't get it. She kept saying, "Tell me again why you
> have to go to the hospital."
>
> Eleanor, 64—consultant

Ann, fifty-nine, a museum curator, made a different choice:

> I didn't tell my parents. I thought it would kill them. They were in their
> eighties. They really wouldn't understand and I didn't want to burden
> them. I had to wear a wig and told my mother that my hair was worn
> out after all those years of coloring it, so I was growing it in without any
> processing.

Dean, sixty-three, a professor, recounted how his parents and
parents-in-law were all in their late eighties and in somewhat
fragile health. He had been planning to visit them all in a few
days when he got the results of the biopsy and so everything was
up in the air—he didn't know how bad it was or what treatment
he was going to choose. He went anyway.

> I really obsessed about how to tell them: When? How much? What
> words? How to minimize their anxiety? Then I realized I was spending
> way too much time worrying about how they might respond, when what
> I needed to do was worry about learning what I needed to know and tak-
> ing care of my own anxiety. I ended up just telling them. Each of them
> reacted in ways I would have never anticipated—really against type. But
> no one got hysterical, and my dad and my mother-in-law were quite
> comforting.

James Cooper, a geriatrician and director of the Memory Disorders Clinic at Washington Hospital Center in Washington, D.C.,
believes that every parent–adult child relationship is unique. He
observes that there is not much research on whether or how you
should tell your parents about your diagnosis. "Unless your parent is demented [suffering from Alzheimer's or a similar disease],"
he says, "I would go by this: What would you want your children
to tell you about their illness? Your parents are grown-ups; they
can take it, and they might even be helpful."

Much of this decision depends on the health of your parents, your relationship with them, where they live, and your assessment of how this might affect them. It may be a good idea to
wait until you have both the diagnosis and treatment plan figured out before you tell them anything. If waiting to find out
more things is hard on you, the uncertainty will be hard on
them.

Telling a Parent about His or Her Own Diagnosis

"We still hear it: 'Don't tell mother she's got cancer.' Families are so odd—the family doesn't want the patient to know, the patient doesn't want the family to know, and the doctor is in the middle. And the person who is sick has all the hope but gets worse," said Paul Wallace, an oncologist and a quality innovator at Kaiser Permanente, in Oakland, California.

Doctors are rarely willing these days to conspire with families to keep a diagnosis from a family member, regardless of their cultural heritage or beliefs. "Withholding information from patients has no legal standing," said Steve Shea, senior associate dean of clinical affairs at Columbia University College of Physicians and Surgeons. "There is a legal construct that says there is a glowing laser line [defining doctors' responsibilities] but it doesn't map onto real people. For example, I take care of people after heart attacks who sometimes have very limited insight. What do we do about telling mentally ill, demented, retarded, and incapacitated individuals about their diagnosis? Physicians try to do this protectively but we have been accused of paternalism—it makes us toss up our hands."

When the family collectively makes a decision to withhold a diagnosis from the member it directly concerns, it means that this person will not have the opportunity to learn about the disease and to make decisions about his or her life and death. Sometimes patients don't want to know or they want to know very little. "I always ask patients what they understand already and then allow them to tell me when they've heard enough, but other people should not make this decision for them," said Karen Antman, of Boston University.

Family members usually withhold information about a diagnosis because they want to protect their loved ones. Culture is a very important determinant of how news of a grave illness is viewed, and the traditional norms from a number of cultures about how illness is treated within families often come smack up against the requirements of modern medicine.

"I found colon cancer in an elderly Chinese man. The whole family was there and they rushed me out of the room. 'He can't know,' they said. I replied that he already knows—he's yellow and losing weight. I had to negotiate with the family. I would have withdrawn as his physician if they had not agreed that he know. This still happens and it requires sensitive conversations. But realistically, people don't overlook the fact that they are in the hospital and have just had twenty tests," said Paul Wallace, of Kaiser Permanente.

"What I tell my patients and their loved ones is, 'What if it was you and all this stuff was happening around you and no one told you what was going on? You'd be angry that people didn't treat you like an adult—that they withheld information that is more critical to you than to anyone in the world.'"

If this doesn't convince you that patients should know their own diagnosis, consider this:

Eliana Horta, a clinical nurse specialist, said, "If I know my own diagnosis, I free other people from the burden of making hard decisions about me. Then I can share a loving relationship with my family without the barriers of secrecy."

Getting a Little Help from Friends and Family

Some people have no trouble asking for help during these first few weeks. They just put the news of their diagnosis out there and assume that help will be forthcoming. And often it is.

> People wanted to be helpful. I don't know how it happened—the kids got to nursery school. People didn't ask. They just swept in and took over car pool and meals.
>
> Terry, 36—foundation executive

But some people experience this time differently. Maybe their friends or acquaintances are not forthcoming with offers. Some people are unaccustomed to needing assistance for almost anything and find it difficult to ask for help.

> It frightens me to be ill because I am alone. It is so hard to ask people when you know you are imposing on their busy schedules. You lose your dignity when you are at your most vulnerable.
>
> Ara, 49—journalist

If you are uncomfortable with the prospect of asking friends or acquaintances for help, but know you need at least a little assistance during this time, even if only to go to doctors' appointments with you, ask yourself: "If I knew someone in this situation, how would I feel about helping them?"

People feel terrible when they hear about what is going on with you. They want to help. Consider giving them something to do. If you need some ideas about how to do this, try this approach:

- List all the people who, when hearing of your diagnosis, said to you, "If there is anything I can do, please let me know." Add the people who might have said that, had the circumstances been right—such as people you like and you know are concerned about you—or would be if they knew what was up. Then add the people whose role it is to help you in various ways, for example, your priest or rabbi and the human resources person at work.

- List all the things you think you need help with now and will need help with in the future: Watch your kids or stay with your ill husband when you have to go get a test done. Accompany you to an appointment with your doctor. Help you research something on the Internet. Pick up some groceries for you. Help you figure out your health insurance. Listen while you talk about how you're feeling about this whole thing.

- See if you can match the people to the tasks. Who would you trust your kids with who might have the time? Who uses their computer to find things out? Whose judgment do you admire? Who would you feel comfortable talking to? Designating one likely person for each task will help.

Then you call the first one and say: "You remember that I was just diagnosed with X and am still figuring out what I am going to do about it. I wondered if you would be able to help me out on something." Then say what it is you need and when. For example, "I have a doctor's appointment next Friday and I find it is better if I don't go alone. I need someone there to take notes to make sure I get all the information I need. Would you be available?"

Or, "I am going through a lot of turmoil about my condition and what I am going to do about it and I need to lay it out and talk it through with someone. I like the way you think and trust your judgment, and was wondering if you'd be willing to have coffee with me and talk sometime this week or next."

It's hard to say these words if you are not used to doing so. You may be surprised that many people are pleased to be asked; they really meant it when they said they would like to help out.

But sometimes the scheduling doesn't work out or, rarely, the person was just being polite and had no intention of helping you.

> You really put your heart on your sleeve when you do this. You can't get all your help from one person. I asked the person who went to the doctor with me to come visit me and she couldn't. My feelings were so hurt. People said, "Oh—I'll do anything you want, please let me do something." I called one of these people to ask her to pick up some milk for my children and she said no. I was devastated.
>
> When I had a lucid moment, I wrote down on index cards everything I thought I needed. So when people asked me, I said, "Take a card." I still got my feelings hurt but it seemed a little less personal and I felt more organized.
>
> Marilyn, 59—minister

If you are uncomfortable asking for help, it is even harder if you have summoned up the energy to ask and the person refuses, especially after they offered to help. But stick with it. If they are not available, ask if they would be willing to accompany you in the future or pick up groceries or go out for coffee. And try not to take it personally; it's not a comment on you or their feeling about you if they are not able or willing to drop what they are doing to help you out.

Move on to the next person on the list.

It's this simple: if you cannot manage all of the responsibilities of keeping your life going and getting the care you need by yourself, you need help. Very few people, sick or well, have the strength to go it alone.

You may be able to hire people to do some of the things you need—deliver groceries, mow the lawn. But the help you need may be beyond your means, may not be available where you live, or may simply not be something you can buy. If not enough people step forward, you must ask. It is not a sign of weakness. You have not lost a popularity contest. It is just how things are right now.

This is an extraordinary crisis and it requires that you do things that you would not ordinarily do to save your own life. You may be disappointed in some of your friends. Move on before you become distracted by this. Right now, ask for help with the things you need.

Putting Out the Fire

"It is as though the house is on fire and everyone in the family grabs a bucket and starts throwing water on the front porch. What about the rest of the house? There is fire in the attic, in the back bedroom," says Teresa Schrader, an internist and medical journalist at Mount Auburn Hospital in Rhode Island.

"Everyone comes to the house or the hospital after work and maintains a vigil, leaving the diagnosed person alone all the rest of the time. This may work for a day or so, while you are absorbing the shock, but believe me, there are many ways of being there for someone you love. If you are the person who talks to your dad about sports, come by or call regularly to do that. If you are the one who is good at doing research on the Internet, take on that task. If you are good with money, offer to keep on top of the bills. Check in daily or more frequently, but divide up the time and the responsibilities. There will be plenty to go around."

Getting a life-altering diagnosis is emotionally exhausting for the person as well as those close to him or her. Let the person with the diagnosis indicate whether she wants company or to be alone, whether she wants to rest or to chat.

There is usually a lot to be done during the time just after someone gets a diagnosis—tests to get scheduled and conducted, information to be gathered and absorbed, appointments to be made, and so on. Let people know how they can help. But remember, it is your life, your diagnosis, and you should be the one whose preferences are honored in dividing up these tasks.

A number of people reported telling the person who everyone assumed would naturally take on key responsibilities that he wasn't the right person for the job, that they wanted someone else to do this. The people who are closest to you may not be the ones you want to accompany you to the doctor and talk through your decisions with. Those closest to you may not be the right person for the job: they may be too upset by the prospect of what is to come to be helpful or there may be someone who has better skills and more knowledge or is better able to interact effectively with doctors, for example. If someone you don't really want around you insists on helping, consider asking them to do a task that doesn't involve much contact with you.

> My sister is a kind of hysterical person and my diagnosis just set her off. I didn't need that, plus a friend who is an unemployed nurse offered to come with me to all my appointments and be the person who watched out for me when I was in the hospital. I told my sister that my friend was going to do this and she felt angry and betrayed. I was sorry to hurt her but I was too upset to take care of her and always be looking out for what was going to make her lose it.
>
> Lara, 44—insurance executive

> I had one friend who really wanted to come to doctors' appointments with me but she was just too upset and teary. This made me even more upset and I finally told her to stay away for a while. I am someone who tends to take care of people and I just couldn't spare the energy to comfort her.
>
> Hannah, 37—teacher

> My mom would have been there in a hot second and she would have given me good emotional support. But I really needed someone there who could understand the complicated medical terms and choices I had to make. So I asked a friend from school to come to appointments. And sometimes my mom came, too.
>
> Lynn, 42—engineer

Families and extended groups of friends vary widely in the way they respond to a health crisis. But remember, everyone is doing the best he or she can. This is an emotional time. Relationships intensify during a crisis. There is anecdotal evidence that good ones get better and bad ones get worse. Kindness, patience, and tolerance will be needed. While things may sometimes get sticky, it is important to keep in sight your shared aim: to figure out how to help you live as well as you can for as long as you can.

CHAPTER 4

Find the Right Doctors and Hospitals

Your aim is to find doctors who treat you with respect, who listen and respond to your concerns, in whose expertise you have confidence, and whom you trust to do their best for you.

No man should entrust himself and his family to any doctor whom he has not carefully judged. Certainly he would never consider allowing any untested artist to paint his portrait.

—Scribonius Largus, pharmacist, First century AD*

LIKE ME, everyone I interviewed for this book had visited doctors throughout the course of their lives, regardless of their overall state of health. Many had regular checkups, sought help from doctors for minor illnesses and quite a few had been diagnosed with chronic conditions—a bad back, gout, arthritis, diabetes, high blood pressure. They had consulted with specialists—cardiologists, endocrinologists, gynecologists—and considered these specialists to be part of their routine health care. In other words, none of us was new to the challenge of getting health care in the United States.

But all of us reported feeling bewildered by the range of doctors we encountered once we were on an urgent mission to respond to our diagnoses: Who are these doctors? What do they know? Which specialists, subspecialists, or sub-subspecialists do I need to consult, why and in which combinations? How do I know which doctors have the expertise to give me the best shot

---

*A. A. Pellegrino, "Humanism and Ethics in Roman Medicine: Translation and Commentary on a Text of Scribonius Largus," in *The Persisting Osler II; Selected Transactions of the American Osler Society*, ed. J. A. Barondes and C. G. Roland, 21–34 (Malabar, Florida: Krieger Publishing Company, 1994).

at getting better? How do doctors communicate with one another about me?

Not knowing the answers to these questions should not embarrass you. You have probably been spending your time engaged with more interesting things. And now, with any luck, you will be able to approach these questions on a need-to-know basis.

Some people are taken in hand early by their own internist or the first specialist they see. This person makes referrals to different specialists he or she knows, may help to coordinate the sequence of consultations and tests, and might even deliver the treatment.

However, many of us find ourselves on our own—either through circumstance or by choice—in identifying doctors to care for us now that we have a devastating diagnosis. This is a kind of odd position to be in. Not only do most of us lack the expertise to evaluate physicians' overall competence when choosing among doctors, but it is also difficult to assess whether our own personal care represents the best clinical medicine can offer.

This chapter provides some facts about physicians in the United States that can help you figure out how much you need to know to feel comfortable with your doctor. It fills in the blanks on the topics that most puzzled the people I interviewed for this book. And it offers different approaches to checking out the expertise and competence of physicians generally and why you might want to look around for the right physicians. It answers common questions people have about how things work with doctors in a situation that is urgent; for example, how to relate to your family practitioner during this time if you have one.

Doctors and nurses comment on how they approach finding physicians for themselves and their families and share what they think might be helpful for patients to know during this difficult period.

Appendix C will guide you on the specifics of finding the doctors who can help determine the treatment and care that is right for you.

The final section of the chapter is about hospitals. Some people have a choice of hospitals, sometimes because they want to go to a hospital that specializes in treating their disease or because they live in a city with many hospitals. If you have a choice of hospitals, take a look at this section for some ideas about how you might approach this decision.

Find Out More about Your Doctor or Not?

A number of people I interviewed were not interested in learning anything about other doctors. They liked and trusted the ones they had. They felt that any time spent checking out the doctors they were already using or searching for additional opinions about their diagnosis or treatment would mean time lost—the disease might get worse during the delay. They were anxious to get started with their treatment.

> I didn't do any research. I believe that when you are told exactly what you have and exactly what the treatment is, you should go with it. I got the exact same opinion twice from really good doctors. I believe you just have to accept your treatment and not get so pumped up.
>
> Clara, 60—administrator

Among that group, there were a few people who had very aggressive diseases that might have been fatal if they had delayed. But this was not true for most.

The majority of the people I interviewed had diseases that needed to be attended to soon—within the next month or two—but their fear made them anxious to come to a decision about doctors and treatments *right now*, so they just ignored the possibility that their current doctor might not be the best one for them or that they should get additional opinions. (See chapter 1, page 6.)

There were, of course, people who dived wholeheartedly into finding the best doctors. They immersed themselves in comparing physicians based on placement in their graduating class, their fellowships, with which medical guru they studied, and the prestige of the journals in which they published. Most of these people were satisfied with the doctors they ultimately chose, but some of them continued to move from doctor to doctor, always finding new doctors who just *might* be better than the ones they currently saw.

What I heard was that, regardless of the objective urgency of one's condition, we each respond differently to the task of finding the right doctor for us. Nevertheless, there are reasons to put some energy into making sure you have the right physician to treat you or to give you additional opinions on your diagnosis.

FOUR REASONS TO GATHER INFORMATION ABOUT A DOCTOR

1. *Medical knowledge is advancing fast.* This means specialists become even more specialized every year and means that doctors have to work hard to stay up-to-date with the latest developments.

There is so much new knowledge about treating some conditions that even specialists who only treat one disease have to constantly read and learn to keep up with innovations in treatment. Some doctors—both specialists and generalists like family doctors—lose interest over time in reading about new treatment approaches in medical journals or going to conferences to learn. Others are cautious about using the latest standards of care until they are well-tested by others. The bottom line is that being treated for a life-altering condition by a doctor who delivers care based on outdated standards can limit your options and reduce your chances of getting the best possible outcome.

2. *The quality of health care in the United States is poorer than most people imagine.* Giving good medical care is challenging to begin with and it is further complicated by rapid changes in knowledge and technology. As I mentioned earlier, a number of studies have recently shown that about half the time, doctors fail to reliably conduct and order tests, prescribe drugs, and otherwise deliver care that has been shown to be effective. Your aim in learning a little about your physicians—and about hospitals—is to increase the likelihood that you will receive care that is based on the best available scientific knowledge about what works.

3. *Experience counts.*

> I liked my colon/rectal surgeon from the moment I met him. I liked him because he was intelligent and professional. He moved methodically in

his examining room—he had done this a thousand times before. He was very efficient in his answering of each of my questions. He had no time for extra talk, but it was obvious that he had a patient's life that was in jeopardy and he wanted to solve the case. I kept listening to his discussions about me with other physicians. He would quickly say, "She's young and healthy, that's on her side."

Maral, 44—writer

There is considerable evidence that the patients of doctors who have conducted a surgical procedure many times or who have treated a relatively rare condition frequently do better than those who are seen by physicians with less experience. Medical treatment relies heavily on a physician's clinical judgment about how to apply new medical advances, and a doctor who has treated many patients with your condition will draw on that experience when working with you to determine your treatment plan.

While it seems this might be an argument for only working with older physicians, it is not. With the increase in specialization it is possible to find young physicians fairly recently out of training who may have extensive experience with only your disease.

4. *Doctors don't do a great job at policing their peers.* Some people find a wall of diplomas in their doctor's office a reassuring sight. And it is, indeed, important that your physician is adequately trained and able to document this training. But this alone may not guarantee that she or he is the right physician for you.

Being a licensed physician means that you can provide any treatment, even though there may be widespread agreement within the profession that certain treatments require additional training. So for example, a family physician could diagnose and treat a tumor in your auditory canal, but chances are that the outcome would be better if a neurologist or neurosurgeon did so. And of course, not all neurologists or all neurosurgeons are equally skilled.

Medicine does a pretty poor job at policing itself against more serious problems. While it is possible to find out which physicians have been disciplined by their state medical board or repeatedly sued for malpractice, this is done on a state-by-state basis and there is nothing to prevent a physician from simply moving to another state.

These considerations may make you uneasy. They are evidence that you may be on your own in finding good doctors. On the other hand, if you have already been referred to a specialist you like by a doctor you know and trust, you may choose to proceed with the physicians you already know.

You want to receive the health care that is right for you, whether that means slowing the progression of a disease, halting it altogether, or making sure that you are comfortable if this is not possible. Your doctor should be the person who has the scientific knowledge and the experience to make sense of your individual situation and risks to treat you.

Taking a little time to gather information about doctors who might treat you is not that difficult and is worthwhile; it can reduce the risk of getting poor-quality care and can increase your confidence that your doctor will use his or her best judgment to find treatments for you that reflect the best available medical science and your own preferences.

Should you choose to seek care from practitioners of alternative medicine, your standards should be no less stringent. You will want to:

- Find practitioners who are well trained, have a solid reputation, and have been certified by a reputable institution.

- Hear good things about this practitioner from a number of people.

- Talk with the practitioner: How many people with your disease has this person treated and what were the outcomes, both positive and negative?

- Know about the treatments, their effectiveness, the possible complications, and the side effects.

- Use laboratory and other markers from medicine to see if the treatment is working.

See chapter 5 for a list of questions to ask about treatment.

"I had an alternative medicine doctor who said, 'Don't look at traditional markers because it will just make you upset,'" said Andrew Robinson, a patient advocate. "When you go into the medical world, it is tough, dour, and stark. Alternative practitioners are warm, optimistic, and hopeful. This is nice but it might not be appropriate in your case. When you are desperate, you will jump through a lot of hoops and you are susceptible to someone who says things that are positive—it just feels better. You really have to check yourself."

Common Questions

Here are some questions that you might have when you first encounter the challenge of finding the right doctors after you have received a bad diagnosis:

What do I expect from my doctor?

I have a friend who looked for a doctor with a good bedside manner but I looked for one who keeps people alive. Who has the best record? I don't care if they are nice. Just smart.

Ann, 59—museum curator

Before you call the physician who treated your neighbor or check online to see which of two possible doctors sounds more qualified, you may want to clarify for yourself what you are looking for because this will influence your search and your decision. Ask yourself what you *expect* from the doctors who you will choose to treat this new condition.

- Are you looking for someone who can deliver a miracle or a cure?

- Are you looking for someone who will assuage your fear and tell you everything is going to be fine?

- How important to you is it that your doctor becomes like a friend, who hugs you and jokes with you and knows about your hobbies?

- How much value do you place in your doctor being competent and responsible?

- Are you looking for a doctor to coordinate your care for this condition or just to address one aspect of it?

Talking about your expectations of your doctor with a family member or trusted friend or writing a list of your expectations can help direct about your search. The best doctors for you are ones who meet your expectations and whose experience, expertise, and intentions you trust. You need to feel that this person is going to care for you in a way that is consistent with your needs.

I can't tell you here—nor can any book or Web site or personal recommendation make the judgment for you—whether you will feel comfortable with any given physician. You need to talk with the doctor and get a sense that you can trust and work with him or her.

"You *have* to develop a trusting relationship with your doctor," said pediatrics nurse leader Shelley McKaye. "If you don't, it's a struggle through the treatment. People are so educated and have so many resources, they no longer are comfortable with the approach, 'Okay, I'll do whatever you say.' Once you decide on your treatment, you have to stop second-guessing your doctors and let their experience and expertise kick in."

Why a specialist or subspecialist?

I feel strongly that one needs to take advantage of the expertise of those who focus on a single disease. I solicited the opinions of several experts and did some background checking and brushed up on current treatments. It is hard to pore over survival curves and think about where I might fall.

Arne, 55—surgeon

The rapid pace of medical research has produced findings that improve the odds that diseases will be discovered earlier in their course and sometimes treated so that people are able to live much longer than they were able to even twenty years ago. Consider HIV/AIDS, for example. In 1986, AIDS was a fatal disease. Now, with the discovery of new drugs and treatments, people can live with it for many years as a chronic condition.

A by-product of this explosion of new knowledge is that there is a lot known about the treatment of many diseases—so much so that, in order to incorporate all the new advances, some physicians focus exclusively on treating single diseases. So, for example, there are surgeons who specialize in treating only colo-rectal cancer, immunologists who treat only HIV/AIDS, neurologists who treat only dementia.

Why is this important to you now? First, because the more frequently a physician has treated a given condition, the more likely it is that her patients will have a good outcome. Second, the sheer volume of new information about treatment for many diseases means that it is difficult for nonspecialists to keep up with new developments. And third, for most serious conditions, there is more than one single treatment. Your treatment will be influenced by the specialty of the physician. Surgeons are more likely to make use of surgery, whereas oncologists, for example, are more likely to recommend chemotherapy.

These are the reasons you have been referred to a specialist in the first place, and they are also reasons you may wish to seek additional opinions from specialist physicians who are real experts in treatment of your condition.

What's the relationship supposed to be between my regular doctor and the specialists who are going to care for me now?

My internist referred me to a specialist for trouble swallowing. I was diagnosed with cancer and treated intensively for about a year. I went back to my internist afterward. He said, "Hey! Looks like you lost a lot of weight, huh?" So I briefly recounted the events of the past year. Having heard it once, he has never brought up the fact that I had had cancer again. It is only now that I am experiencing problems as a result of my cancer treatment that I realize that my internist would have benefited from talking to my oncologist and my oncologist would have benefited from knowing about my medical history.

Jaime, 47—musician

If you have a doctor who has treated you over the years and is familiar with you, this new diagnosis will put your relationship on a different footing. In all likelihood, this physician will not treat you. Rather, you will need or want to consult with one or more specialists who are expert in treating your condition.

If your regular doctor or nurse practitioner has been involved in your diagnosis—in other words, if you first went to her with your symptoms and she referred you to the specialist—the specialist may communicate your diagnosis to your doctor. It is less likely that the specialist will continue to communicate with your regular doctor after this, however. Then it is up to you.

If, however, you were not referred to a specialist by your regular doctor, he or she will not know that you have this condition. It often happens that once patients start consulting with specialists, their regular physician—whether he or she is a family doctor or internist or gynecologist—fades out of the picture. But there are several important reasons why you will want to involve your regular doctor.

First of all, your regular physician may be willing to sit down with you and review your diagnosis and test results to help you understand your options. Particularly if you have had a long-standing relationship, this physician can combine medical expertise with some knowledge of you personally as you evaluate care options. Make an appointment and do this in person if possible.

Second, if your regular doctor has known you for a while and is familiar with your history, she can talk to your treating physicians to make sure they know about events in your medical history or your individual sensitivities that may bear on your treatment.

And, third, your regular physician cares what happens to you. While she may be very busy, you are still her patient and she wants you to do as well as possible. Keeping her in the loop will help her stay invested in your progress and will help ensure that she will be able to continue to care for you effectively in the future.

Internist/medical journalist Teresa Schrader suggests that you may want to tell your regular doctor about your diagnosis. Ask her, "What part of this can you help me with? I don't want to waste your time or my time or overstep your expertise as I work with specialists to be treated for this new condition. But what about my other health needs: my arthritis, for example. Will you be in touch with me? Or do you just want me to check in?"

Regardless of whether you have a regular doctor, remember that you are not your disease. Specialists treat specific diseases. Regardless of the course of the specific disease you are so concerned about right now, you still may need a doctor to care for the occasional ear infection, sprained ankle, or migraine headache. Your specialist is not that doctor. Once in the midst of one of my own health crises I complained to my gynecological oncologist about recurring headaches and he retorted, "That's not my body part."

Also, while minor conditions may fade into the background during this very stressful time, it is important not to minimize or neglect other health concerns. If you have diabetes, for example, and have just been diagnosed with Parkinson's disease, it may be difficult to maintain your usual care with eating and medication because of the stress.

How should I communicate with my doctors?

Talking with your doctor—and being certain you are listened to—is a very important part of working together closely over time. At the point when you have just been diagnosed, you may be seeing a number of different specialists. Here are few important pointers about talking with doctors during this early period.

If you don't understand something, ask. Even if it's the answer to a question you just asked—tell the doctor you didn't understand. You need to understand the answer because you need to make important decisions that are based, at least in part, on this information.

Not understanding something and asking about it does not mean that you are stupid. It means that the doctor either doesn't understand your question or has not been able to use language and examples that are sufficiently clear. The doctor knows that your diagnosis has put a tremendous strain on you and that it is difficult to take in complicated information when you are under so much stress. It is part of the doctor's job to make sure you *do* understand.

Often, however, doctors are rushed or use words and ideas that are technical and unfamiliar to nonprofessionals. It is also the case that, because doctors live day in and day out thinking about this condition, they tend to forget how little you know when you just find out about it. Sometimes they also err on the side of overestimating your sophistication about medicine and don't explain things fully.

It took me a couple of bad illnesses before I started to ask about everything I didn't understand. I used to think my doctors would think I was stupid and was embarrassed to ask. Then I realized that they were ready to explain, but I needed to tell them when I was confused; otherwise they assumed that I understood everything.

If questions occur to you after your appointment, write them down. If you can't wait to get the answer—not knowing is making you too anxious—wait until you have two or three questions, then call the office and ask the nurse whether she can answer the questions or whether she thinks the doctor should return your call. Take notes on the answers. If you don't understand something, ask about it. Some physicians are willing to communicate by e-mail or fax.

Don't be surprised if your doctor doesn't know the answers to all your questions or uses words like "maybe" and "might" and "try." Medicine is based on probability. There is a probability that your symptoms and the tests conducted so far mean that you might have a specific disease but it is not certain at this point. Having a given disease may increase the probability of death but it doesn't guarantee it within a specific amount of time. The answers to both questions depend on a wide range of factors, some of which are obvious—for example, the stage of the disease, your age, sex, and medical history. Others are not obvious—for example, other test results, your genetic makeup, and your history of exposure to environmental toxins. Your doctor may be able to provide a rough guess as to the answer for many questions but will not be able to reassure you that this will certainly take place on a specific timetable.

"Just because your doctor doesn't tell you what to do doesn't mean he or she is not competent. Some patients are very proactive. But most people cannot find the mental model of their condition without the help of their doctor. For some people, when [the] doctor doesn't tell them what to do, they think he is wacky— or when [the] doctor admits uncertainty, [they] think he is incompetent," explained a physician executive for a health plan.

Most doctors will provide clear guidance about what you need to do to confirm your diagnosis—what tests you need to evaluate your circumstances, for example—and will recommend where you have the tests done. They may or may not suggest that you get another opinion. But often they will lay out choices about your treatment and care rather than telling you what to do.

As medicine advances, there may be treatment choices that only you can make, that is, the outcomes of the different approaches are statistically the same but the timing and side effects may differ greatly. Since you will be the one living with the risks, the outcomes, and the side effects, only you can make these decisions (see chapter 10).

Ideas from Physicians about Finding the Right Doctors

Physicians I spoke to were generally in favor of visiting academic medical centers (usually medical centers associated with universities) to confirm a diagnosis and a treatment plan.

For example, Michael Zinner, chief of surgery at Brigham and Women's Hospital in Boston, said, "I have a bias for teaching hospitals—I bring the bias to the table. I think institutions that do credible research as well as train the next generation have a special responsibility. But only twenty percent of the care in the country is delivered there."

Some people get the benefit of a specialty hospital or academic medical center by consulting physicians there about a treatment plan and then asking for a referral closer to home for the treatment itself. "Physicians in research hospitals often know the players in their region and they know whether they are good or not. Specialists at academic medical centers are busy and don't want patients sticking to them. They are willing to make a referral and it doesn't mean they are abandoning you," said Zinner.

Ned Cassem, a psychiatrist at Massachusetts General Hospital in Boston, added, "Getting a doctor who is the best researcher in bladder cancer means you get a good researcher, it doesn't mean you get a good doctor. I have on my door a plaque that says 'A good doctor takes care of the disease; a great doctor takes care of the patient.'"

"It is a myth that there is only one doctor, one specialist for you. Not everyone who trains at a teaching hospital stays there," said Robert Krasner, an internist on the faculty at New York University School of Medicine and former attending physician in the U.S. Capitol. "There are official and unofficial satellites and they put out many fellows every year, not all of whom go to other academic settings. They are in practice all over the country."

Does this mean you need to travel far from home for your treatment? "It depends on where you are. If you have a really unusual condition, you may have to. But common diseases are common, even though they may be life-threatening and you probably can be treated well close to home," said Krasner.

And when a physician looks for a doctor to treat himself or his family?

> I am looking for expertise, experience, and good judgment to sort through complicated information, to balance what's known with what's not and the ability to make a decision in the absence of complete data. I want her to love what she does and be excited, not threatened, by new advances. I want her to have good staff who shares that enthusiasm. I want access—I want my calls returned; if I have a medical question, I don't want it answered by a secretary. I want to know that my doctor is communicating with others on the team. I want my privacy respected— I don't want family members or other patients to know my business. And finally, I want my doctor to take me and my concerns seriously.
>
> Marisa Weiss—oncologist, president and founder of
> Breastcancer.org

> I want someone who will listen to me—will be compassionate and take the time to understand my situation. When I get my big life-changing diagnosis, I want a physician who will *be there*, not someone who is off giving a paper in Paris or taking care of a princess somewhere. I want a doctor who will call me back, who is knowledgeable, sympathetic, willing to listen to what I want and will help me figure out what I want because I could be overwhelmed—so this person will help me draw on my own experience to do it. So unless I have a really exotic diagnosis, you won't see me with a big-name guy at a big-name hospital. They are interested in really complicated, esoteric diseases. I want someone who is interested in treating my garden-variety prostate cancer or whatever, not someone who is bored with something that for them is everyday but for me is a threat to my life.
>
> William Popick—family physician and former chief medical
> officer of Aetna

This is what I want as a patient and what I think you want: someone who will say to you, "I don't know if this treatment will be helpful—when we look at the literature what we get is the range and the mean. I can't tell where in the range you will fall. This therapy has been helpful in some people in your situation. There is an opportunity to intervene and you and I will do this together. I will provide the best I can and try to get you the best there is. We will repeatedly evaluate. We won't make the total decision now. I will mobilize with you. I will be with you. And if this doesn't work—we will try something different."
Jeremiah Barondess—president, New York Academy of Medicine, and professor emeritus of Clinical Medicine at Cornell University

Six Things That Doctors Want Patients to Know about Doctors

1. *We know how hard it is for you to hear this news.*

Physicians I interviewed know that this is a terribly difficult time for you. They have, in the course of their careers, delivered bad news many times. Some say it is difficult when they don't know a person because they aren't sure what kind of support he has to help him absorb this information. Others say that it's hard to give bad news to patients they have known for a long time—that it's like telling a member of their own family.

"While people vary in their abilities to respond, *no one* really takes in the whole thing (nor should they be expected to) at one time. People feel the need to be chipper, to be brave for their family. This is a terrific load and it takes a lot of getting used to. No one finds it easy. It is my responsibility—the doctor's—to help the patient knit together the tasks," said Jeremiah Barondess.

2. *We don't know the answer to the question "When?"*

The doctors I interviewed reported that patients and their loved ones always want to know the answer to this question—when will I know? When will I feel better? When will I get out of the hospital? When will I die?

For the most part, doctors simply don't know the answer to these questions, which is not a reason not to ask them. Medical knowledge is based on risk, which means, for example, that re-search might show that 60 percent of patients with a certain di-agnosis who receive a certain treatment will be disease–free in five years. But research doesn't tell, and doctors can't know, whether you will be in the 60 percent. You just must be prepared not to get definite answers.

Because there are so many factors that influence your condi-tion and your treatment, it is difficult, if not irresponsible, for a doctor to promise certain outcomes.

3. We are only part of your health-care experience and hope you will recognize that there are other parts we don't control.

People with devastating diagnoses often quickly develop intense relationships with their physicians, but tend to forget that the physicians work in—and are dependent upon—a network of related organizations that dictate what can and cannot be done. Depending on where he or she works, your doctor may not have any influence, for example, on how frequently the examination room is cleaned, how appointments are made, whether test re-sults are entered into your chart, or how you are charged for the services provided.

I asked a group of physicians at a major teaching hospital if I could tell readers of this book that, to ensure they got copies of test results, they should ask the office staff to photocopy them. This made those doctors hoot with laughter. "What office staff? Tell them to follow us to the photocopy machine and we'll do it ourselves!"

This does not mean that you shouldn't expect competence and high–quality service from your doctor and from the practice, clinic, or hospital. Rather, it means that your physician shares re-sponsibility with others—and with the institution—for your care.

4. We know it is burdensome for people to have to find and evaluate physicians, particularly after receiving a diagnosis of a serious condition.

It used to be easier for patients. Doctors made recommenda-tions and patients followed them. Not any more. But doctors know that many people find it burdensome to have to make their own decisions and judgments about the knowledge and skills of doctors that they know little about. The doctors I talked with felt that they are generally pretty good judges of their colleagues' expertise but also want to caution patients that doctors maintain social and personal ties with other physicians that sometimes interfere with their judgment about their colleagues' competence.

Every single doctor I interviewed recommended getting at least one additional opinion to confirm a serious diagnosis and treatment plan before going forward. This is pretty compelling.

5. *We often see a patient for only an episode of care and thus miss the full story of his condition and how it affects his or her life.*

Specialists are specialists because they focus on one small aspect of human health all day, every day. A radiation oncologist will see twenty patients a day but only for the period during which their treatment calls for radiation. One by one, each patient moves on to surgical or medical oncologists, who also only see her for the period where that kind of treatment is relevant.

This is what you want in a specialist: someone who knows everything about one critical aspect of your treatment. But that means they can't allow themselves to be concerned with other aspects of your illness.

Some patients have specialists who stick with them and coordinate their care as they move from doctor to doctor. But many of us do not, leaving us feeling as if no one is in charge or watching out for us, particularly when all the standard treatments have been exhausted.

If this describes your situation, you may want to ask one of your specialists if she will act in this role, or ask your internist or family physician to do so. If neither of these is possible, you may want to seek an internist who can stick with you and make sure all available information is in one place to help you make decisions. (See page 68.)

6. *Sometimes life intrudes.*

Physicians recounted their regret at the times when their professional demeanor slipped in front of patients. Caring for a demented mother at home, tending a sick child, going through a painful divorce, having an argument with a colleague just before walking into the examining room—all these influence physicians' abilities to give their full attention to the patient in front of them.

Those I interviewed made two important points about this. First, they wanted to remind patients that a doctor's brusqueness or distraction is probably not directed at the patient personally. And second, apart from the assaults of everyday life, physicians' personalities span the full range of the general population. But all of them agreed: There is no excuse for incompetence or rudeness.

Doctors I interviewed fully endorsed the idea that people should not force themselves to work with doctors they do not feel listen to them or respect them or whose abilities they doubt. They urged patients to find doctors they like and trust.

"From the patient's perspective, I am probably the only oncologist you are ever going to have, but for me you are just another patient. Because of this, I have to constantly remind myself that every word I say matters deeply to you," said Paul Wallace, of Kaiser Permanente.

Your Strategy for Finding the Right Doctor

Many people I talked to described themselves as being in the dark about how to tell whether a doctor had the right expertise and experience to treat them. And there *are* pieces of information that will help you get some sense of these qualities.

Appendix C provides an outline of two approaches for checking out a doctor's background. It includes a list of questions and suggests where you might find the answers. One of these approaches is basic—it assumes that you are comfortable with the referrals you have and just want to independently confirm what you know about the doctors in whose hands you are placing your care.

The other is a more comprehensive approach to identifying and checking out doctors who may have the right expertise and approach for you. It requires a more significant investment of time and resources to answer all the questions, and assumes that you need a fuller palette of information to feel comfortable.

Neither approach guarantees competence or excellence, but

both offer you ways to increase the likelihood that you will find a physician who can fulfill your expectations.

Are You Choosing among Hospitals?

Usually, people make the choice of a physician to care for them without considering his or her hospital affiliation. But in the case of serious sudden illness, hospital choice sometimes trumps physician choice. For example, you hear about people who seek care at the Mayo Clinic or the Cleveland Clinic on the assumption that the medical team that will be assembled for them at these comprehensive, full-service institutions will be able to expertly handle whatever condition they are bringing in the door.

Similarly, some people approach care at a hospital affiliated with a medical school in the belief that physicians who also conduct research will be more likely to be aware of the current standard of care and will also know of promising new advances.

The news coverage of studies showing that the quality of health care received and the high number of medical errors committed differs widely among hospitals, has also raised public awareness about making a choice of hospitals instead of passively accepting a physician's recommendation.

That said, the science of hospital evaluation in terms that are meaningful for patients is still at a fairly early point in its development. "While on the one hand there's a lot more available to the public than there was ten years ago—for example, there is some online hospital performance information, the reality is that its still pretty primitive, particularly relative to the diagnosis of a catastrophic health event," according to Carol Cronin, a consultant on consumer health-care information. Not all hospitals are willing to participate in evaluation, and many of the measures of quality that are tracked are of little interest to consumers or are reported in ways that are not useful to decision-making.

If, however, you *are* planning to find your doctor to treat this diagnosis based on your choice of hospital, or your doctor has admitting privileges in more than one hospital, there are four general considerations to keep in mind:

First, it is important that the hospitals you are considering participate in your health plan or accept Medicare or Medicaid. Hospital care is very expensive—even more so if you are uninsured. If the hospital does not take your insurance or you have no insurance, ask for printed rates for the procedures you expect to have done. Some uninsured people have been known to negotiate a rate in advance; that is, bargain effectively for a cash discount. More typically, however, the uninsured pay higher rates than insurance companies have negotiated. Some hospitals offer payment through an interest-free installment plan. (See chapter 8 about the financial aspects of a serious diagnosis.)

Second, find out if the hospitals you are considering deliver good-quality care and make efforts to avoid medical errors. The best objective way to assess that a given hospital does so is if it adheres to a common standard and has been accredited by the Joint Commission on Accreditation of Healthcare Organizations. You can do this by contacting JCAHO at 630-792-5800 or www.jcaho.org.

This means that the hospital not only has devoted resources to insuring that the way they deliver health care meets these standards, but is also willing to be evaluated on the effectiveness of those efforts and to make the results available to the public. Note that "physicians rarely have a clue about the quality performance of their own hospitals or how the hospitals in which they have privileges compare with others," says Cronin.

Third, you will want to see how your choice of hospitals stacks up against one another. The Medicare program produces a Web site (www.hospital compare.hhs.gov/) that allows you to view how a given hospital performs on delivering care that meets evidence-based standards and to compare the performance of that hospital with the others you are considering. This Web site provides information about aspects of health care for specific conditions (heart failure, heart attack, and pneumonia) and some crosscutting issues, such as surgical infection and patient experience.

Fourth, the way you can judge whether a given hospital is right for you is if the medical and nursing staff has experience treating the condition you have. This information is a little harder to come by. About half the states currently track this information. You can contact your state's health department to see if yours does. In some cases, the JCAHO information will capture a bit of a hospital's track record on specific conditions. The best sources of such data, however, are private Web sites maintained by health plans and employers. If you don't regularly use your health plan's Web site, call the toll-free customer service number on the back of your card and ask if it sponsors an online tool for comparing hospitals' track records in treating certain conditions.

The point here is, of course, that there is evidence that the more experience a hospital team has performing a specific surgery or caring for a certain disease, the better the health outcomes for such patients.

From a more practical perspective, you will want to consider how far the various hospitals are from your home. Most patients and even most hospitals these days recommend having a family member or friend with you for as much of the time as possible. Adding a long drive or plane trip to the physical and emotional task of caring for someone in the hospital may figure into your calculations.

Many serious diagnoses lead to surgery or other debilitating treatments. Even after successful treatment, you might experience significant weakness or functional loss related to your medical situation. Consider asking in advance how rehabilitation services would be handled if they are necessary. Some general hospitals have associated acute inpatient rehabilitation facilities (IRFs); some IRFs are independent of general hospitals. Such acute rehabilitation care might be the right choice for your needs, and sometimes subacute rehab units or skilled nursing facilities (SNFs) are more appropriate for an individual's situation. Often, people are well enough to get any necessary therapy services on an outpatient basis. Either way, you can give yourself the best chance of a full recovery by working with your doctor—or getting referred to a board-certified specialist in physical medicine and rehabilitation—to think about whether, what kind and where rehabilitation services might help. You can check out the accreditation status of any facility offering rehabilitation services to give you confidence about the standards the facility meets.

Knowing whether the hospital has a good social work department is another thing you may inquire about, especially if your condition is one that will require rehabilitation or home health-care arrangements or a change in insurance status. Ask what services the social work department provides.

CHAPTER 5

Gather Expert Opinions about Your Diagnosis and Treatment

The aim of seeking additional opinions is to have confidence that you are going to receive the treatment for your condition that meets your needs and preferences and that will give you the best possible outcome.

When I told my doctor that I was getting another opinion, the doctor said, "What, you don't believe me? No one will treat you at this point in time for this illness." I said that I thought it made sense that since I have a serious disease that I should get at least one additional opinion about what to do. He finally gave me two names and said, "I'd like to hear what they say."

Manuel, 62—real estate investor

I WAS MEETING WITH my newly acquired oncologist and surgeon to schedule an operating room date the day after a routine screening test discovered a dangerous precancerous condition. I thought I could fit major abdominal surgery into my busy schedule four months later. I have responsibilities, after all; people who depend on me, a job, plus I have theater tickets. The doctors countered with, "We think four weeks is the longest you should wait, not four months," thus taking a bite out of the fragile conviction that I didn't really need to be upset by the surprising state of this body part with which I had, until the previous day, only the vaguest acquaintance.

Well, okay. I guess this is more serious than I thought if there is this kind of urgency. I'm ready. I'll do whatever you say, I thought. You are the experts: you know the risks of waiting. I want to get this settled quickly.

And then I froze. I heard my husband casually say, "Could you please give us the pathology report? We'd like to get some other opinions." And the oncologist shot back without missing a beat, "We've already talked about it here among ourselves. You won't find anyone who will disagree with us."

My first thought was, "Who am I to doubt them? They all agree, after all."

Simultaneously, I was thinking, "What if these doctors are angry that we have questioned their judgment? Will they refuse to treat me now? If I continue with them, will they somehow punish me for my lack of confidence in them?"

And my rational self was chirping away: "What if there are alternatives to this surgical cure? This is so sudden and seems so radical and life-altering. How can I commit to this course of action based on the little I know now about what is wrong with me? How can these doctors ask me to go along with this plan when I just learned of this yesterday?"

Well, we got some additional opinions and my oncologist was right: all of the other experts agreed. We went ahead with her original plan and I feel confident that it was the right one, though I remain chastened by my initial passive acceptance of the first treatment that was offered. It is tough to question your doctor when you feel she holds your life in her hands.

Why Should I Consider Seeking Additional Opinions?

Deciding on a course of treatment that is appropriate for your diagnosis and that takes into account your personal preferences and aims may require consulting with a number of physicians.

The notion of getting a second opinion still occupies a prominent place in the minds of both patients and doctors. Yet it is rare these days for someone with a serious diagnosis to be treated exclusively by one physician. Diseases influence different systems within the body, requiring that additional expertise be brought to bear. For example, a neurologist and an orthopedist might be consulted about a back injury, and treating it could require a surgeon or an anesthesiologist in addition.

So the question for you is not about whether you should seek other opinions but, rather, what professional knowledge can be brought to bear on your condition to ensure that you have the right treatment for you?

The idea of getting additional opinions about your diagnosis and treatment has undoubtedly been raised—by you, a friend, a family member, or even your doctor. For many people like me, the desire to make decisions and have a plan for action in place is so strong that they decide arbitrarily that their current doctor and the treatment she has recommended is just fine. "Let's just get started!" Others, however, set out to consult with any doctor anywhere in the world who might offer some obscure or novel treatment that will improve their prospects.

Despite these differences, all of us are looking for the same thing: the sudden uncertainty we face is devastating and we want to act to end it. We just have different strategies for doing so. But there are dangers inherent in each one.

Those who decide not to check their diagnosis and treatment with at least one additional physician take a risk that they will not receive state-of-the-science care. As noted in chapter 4, there is considerable evidence that doctors deliver care that is based on the best available evidence only about half the time. And this is for fairly common diseases with straightforward treatments. Imagine, then, what this means about care for less common diseases whose treatments are less studied! By checking to make sure you will receive the current standard of care, you can reassure yourself that you are getting the right treatment for you.

Those who seek opinion after opinion, hoping to find agreement about what to do next also take on additional risks by delaying their treatment by gathering so much information that they become immobilized and unable to make a decision. One physician likened this process to her husband's plan to take an entire day to choose a new television set. "He seems to think that if he asks enough questions that he can reduce the risks of buying the wrong TV to zero." Similarly, no amount of questioning different doctors can promise 100 percent odds that a treatment will work.

Taking either strategy to the extreme is dangerous but you could drive a truck through the middle ground: How many opinions are enough to make sure I am getting the best for me but not so many that I am wasting precious time and money? So before you make a quick decision about getting—or not getting—additional expert advice, consider what is known about seeking medical opinions and some of the factors that might influence how you proceed.

This chapter answers practical questions about how to approach this task:

- Under what circumstances should I definitely seek other expert opinions?

- How should I approach getting another opinion?

- How do I tell my doctor I want to consult other experts?

- How do I actually go about getting other opinions?

  — How much do I have to be involved?

  — Which doctor?

  — Does insurance cover this?

  — What do I tell the consulting physician's office staff?

  — What should I expect of the opinion?

- How do I make sense of what I learn?

I was surprised by my own reluctance to seek another opinion for fear of antagonizing my diagnosing physician. Since then, I have talked with people who described how they approached the problem of consulting other doctors about what to do while still in shock from getting their bad medical news:

> I couldn't take in any more information. Just knowing I have MS was enough. What good would more information do? I was tempted, though, to keep looking until I found a doctor who said, "Hey! Nothing wrong with you! You just need more sleep."
>
> Chris, 38—physician

> I see my doctor at Rotary every week. If I don't take his advice, he is going to think I don't trust his professional judgment. It would be embarrassing for us both and would end our professional and personal relationship, I'm sure.
>
> Greg, 70—retired lawyer

I couldn't take the time to schedule appointments with other physicians. Not knowing what was going to happen next was unbearable. I was willing to do anything just to have it resolved, just to be doing something rather than just anticipating more bad news, the next sign that something is terribly wrong.

Lee, 42—architect

I had the names of the specialists who treat this condition from six academic medical centers around the country and I went to see every one of them before I even began to consider what I was going to do.

Sharon, 57—university dean

Under What Circumstances Should I Definitely Seek Additional Expert Opinions?

Every doctor, every nurse, and almost every patient I talked with agreed that in this day and age, getting additional opinions about treatment for a life-changing medical diagnosis is critically important.

That said, there are also many diagnoses for which additional opinions are really not necessary because there is only one treatment and it is standard, for example, for diabetes or basal cell skin cancer.

In the few studies on this topic, people reported seeking additional opinions when:

- They wanted more information about their condition or treatment

- They were dissatisfied with their relationship with the doctor, particularly with regard to communication

- They felt they were treated badly

- They thought they would have received better care if they were of a different race

- They felt the treatment they were receiving did not improve their health enough to participate fully in work, school, or other activities

Conventional wisdom says that there are four criteria for which you should seek additional opinions if your situation meets one of the following criteria.

1. *You feel that your doctor has treated you badly.*

If you have just received a really serious diagnosis and your doctor proposes to treat you, you will probably be seeing a lot of him or her in the next couple of months. This person must be someone you can trust, who will talk with you so that you understand your choices, who you think is completely competent to care for you and whom you believe has your best interests in mind.

People vary in their expectations about the communications skills of their doctors—and have a variety of preferences about the kinds of relationships they wish to have. Do you want your doctor to act as a partner? An advisor? A technical consultant?

You may be willing to put up with a physician's bad bedside manner and stinginess with information as long as you are confident about his technical skills. Or it may be important for you to have a good personal relationship with your doctor and to like and trust his manner.

> The doctor who diagnosed me gave me the bad news about my biopsy over the phone—and then asked me if I really wanted to hear this on the phone. She may be a famous doctor, but this was so inconsiderate—and I responded so badly—I didn't feel I could trust her to care for me. I got an opinion from a doctor at another hospital who spent an hour going over my x-rays with me talking about my options. He was kind and understood how alone I felt making these decisions and I knew I wanted him to do my surgery.
>
> Rena, 39—personal trainer

Your relationship with your doctor is a matter of personal preference. And it is absolutely legitimate to consult other physicians until you find one in whom you have confidence to provide the best treatment for you. See chapter 4 for a discussion of this idea.

2. Your doctor has little experience treating your condition.

Patients tend to do better when they are treated by physicians who are thoroughly familiar with a specific disease and its treatment. This is true whether you have a relatively common condition for which there are many advances in treatment but which your doctor doesn't see very often (breast cancer, for example) or a rare condition with which he or she has no experience.

There is considerable evidence that patients treated by doctors who specialize in a single disease and its treatment do better. The saying "practice makes perfect" makes intuitive sense when applied to medical diagnosis and treatment, especially given the speed of new developments in the treatment of many life-threatening conditions.

Hospitals affiliated with medical schools are more likely to have specialists on staff who focus only on your condition and who are in touch with research scientists all over the world who are studying it. You may not ultimately choose to be treated by these doctors, but they may be willing to consult with your own physician by telephone about your care in the future. This is particularly important for those who have rare conditions or who do not live close to a medical center.

> My internist diagnosed my Parkinson's disease, and even though I trust him and know he's seen a lot Parkinson's over the years, I'm pretty sure he's not up on all the latest pharmaceutical research. I wanted to be seen by someone who only thinks about this disease and can tease out which are Parkinson's symptoms and which are heart failure symptoms.
>
> Allan, 75—psychiatrist

3. Your diagnosis is uncertain or borderline.

When looking at the same slides of cancer cells, physicians' observations can vary. Studies that compare a first opinion of a surgical pathologist with a second opinion, even at major academic medical centers, find that there are differences between the two readings that influence diagnosis and treatment of some types of cancer. A report in the journal *Cancer* in the fall of 2005 noted that about 12 percent of U.S. cancer patients are initially misdiagnosed leading to repeat testing, treatment delays, increased health-care costs, and considerable patient anxiety. Changes in diagnosis occur more frequently in borderline conditions, in the early stages of a disease, or in conditions where it is difficult to tell when the tissue irregularity crosses the line to represent malignancy.

If you have been diagnosed based on a pathology report and it does not give a definitive diagnosis or if you have a rare form of your disease it is advisable to seek other pathology opinions.

> Even if your disease isn't all that rare, you may very well benefit from finding someone with a special interest in your cancer. My kind of leukemia is not really rare but it is not exactly common, either. But in my experience, many patients with this kind of leukemia do not get the latest and greatest treatment.
>
> Noam, 38—retail clerk

There are other conditions for which the tests are ambiguous: Parkinson's disease, Alzheimer's disease, ALS, lupus, and multiple sclerosis, for example, depend on multiple indicators, some of which may not agree with one another and that can only be resolved over time as other symptoms develop. The impact of a tentative diagnosis of any one of these diseases is devastating, first because of the prognosis and, second, because it often takes a long time until the diagnosis is confirmed.

> I waited six excruciating months for the symptoms to develop into enough to be identifiable as ALS. I knew there was something wrong but the condition just didn't manifest itself in a definitive way. I was torn between wanting to believe that if my internist couldn't find anything that I was okay and thinking that a different kind of doctor could figure it out. I had to force myself to see specialists.
>
> Raphael, 38—designer

It is important to note, however, that in many cases, test results are clear and there is widespread agreement about both diagnosis and treatment. You may be able to find a physician to give you a different opinion, but you will have to search far and wide for one. Hypertension, diabetes, asthma, heart failure, non-bleeding peptic ulcer, and basal cell skin cancer all fall into this category. Although some people are devastated to learn they have these diseases, others do not experience these diagnoses as life-altering, just inconvenient and something to be managed.

Of course there are borderline cases even with these conditions and there are special considerations (the presence of another acute disease, or impending death, for example) that can provoke uncertainty about whether and how to treat them.

4. *You have been told by your physician that "there is nothing we can do."*

The abolition of hope by a physician is a sin for which there is no absolution.
Jeremiah Barondess, New York Academy of Medicine

Occasionally people are told there is nothing to be done about their condition—there is no treatment available. Sometimes this happens when a disease is very far along in its course and when the disease has no known cure.

Always when a physician makes such a remark, it shows cruelty and a lack of imagination on the part of the physician about how the patient, family, and friends might hear those words. Consider the alternative:

Our doctor was very straightforward that my husband's disease was fatal and that it could not be cured. But he said it could be treated. That was incredibly comforting to both of us.

Hope, 69—archivist

While it is true that many diseases cannot be cured, it is never true that there is nothing to be done. Even when the prognosis is very bad, a physician can refer the patient to a pain management specialist who can provide treatment to reduce discomfort or to a clinical nurse specialist, for example, who can help develop a plan to manage the symptoms of progressive dementia.

There is always the slight chance that an error has been made. For example, although errors in reading pathology reports are rare, they do happen. In addition, different physicians have different views of what is possible. Some physicians are more up-to-date on treatments than others. The same tumor may appear inoperable to one surgeon but operable to another. And finally, exploring ways to live as well as possible with a disease that cannot be cured or treated is worth the effort.

As discussed in chapter 4, even with an unambiguous diagnosis, treatment recommendations vary by profession, institution, and geographic region. Given the same symptoms and pathology, for example, where you live could influence whether your doctor will recommend a hysterectomy. Similar variations have been documented for tonsillitis, prostate and breast cancers, and a number of other conditions.

Physicians view problems through the lens of their training. A surgeon may stress the necessity of surgery to remove a tumor, regardless of how advanced in age the person may be, whereas a geriatrician may be more likely to focus on quality of life as an important criterion.

If after reading this far you are still not interested in getting at least one additional opinion, ask yourself:

- Am I satisfied that my doctor has had lots of experience diagnosing and treating my particular disease?

- Am I positive there are no important or clearly preferable alternatives to undergoing this treatment and experiencing its long-term effects?

- Did this doctor communicate to me exactly what the diagnosis is and what it means? Do I feel comfortable asking him or her questions?

- Am I anxious about discovering that there may be alternative treatments and that I'll have to decide between them?

If you answered yes to the first three questions, then you are probably going to stick with the doctor and plan you have in hand.

If you answered yes to all the questions but your proposed treatment will produce an irrevocable change and you have a little lingering uncertainty about it, then you really should get another opinion. You can bring that opinion back to your first doctor, who will discuss the options with you. Physicians *want* their patients to be convinced they are getting the best treatment because such patients are more likely to follow recommendations and thus may have a better outcome.

But if you answered no to any one of these questions, you may want to weigh the trade-offs between the comfort of a quick resolution (having your next steps laid out clearly right now) and seeking additional opinions. The shock of a life-threatening diagnosis sometimes upsets our normal risk-assessment abilities, making it difficult to come to a firm decision. This is a good time to talk about your thinking with your primary care doctor or internist, a family member, or a friend who can help you sort out whether and how you want to get more expert advice about your condition and its treatment.

How Should I Approach Gathering Expert Opinions?

It helps to approach seeking opinions about your diagnosis and treatment with the attitude that every person and institution you contact has the same goal: to provide you with high quality care that will give you the best outcome and the least discomfort.

Even if you aren't sure whether you need or want other opinions, interact with your diagnosing doctor as though you anticipate getting one. Ask your doctor to tell you exactly what the problem is and to write down the diagnosis, its description, and the technical words so you can look them up. Ask him or her to draw you a picture and ask for a photocopy of the pathology report, radiology report, and/or the blood work.

Here are some questions you can ask to make sure you have enough information to make your decision about seeking another opinion—and to compare opinions should you choose to seek additional advice.

When you talk to your doctor about your *diagnosis*, ask these questions:

1. *"How is this diagnosis generally made?"*

Ask your doctor to educate you about your condition. You are not making an accusation about his or her skills; rather, you are curious and need to understand the situation better. You want to know what tests and clinical assessments went into the diagnosis.

If you decide to get another opinion, this will tell you which laboratory tests, x–rays, and pathology reports you will need to provide and what other information ("you have enlarged lymph nodes") is critical for the next physician to know.

2. *"How certain are you about this diagnosis?"*

Your doctor may not express this as a probability value, but rather may say something along the lines of, "You satisfy all five of the diagnostic criteria," or "We're not sure, but it's better to be safe than sorry."

Remember, ambiguous or borderline diagnoses are a signal to get another opinion.

3. *"Could these symptoms be caused by a different disease? Could this be something else?"*

You are asking about the differential diagnosis—how your doctor distinguished condition X from condition Y. Asking this may prompt your doctor to consider other diagnoses she may have overlooked and it will help you to understand some of the important elements of your condition.

4. *"Is this a rare condition or a fairly common one? How often do you treat patients with this condition?"*

As noted, there is lots of evidence that familiarity breeds expertise in medicine. Think of the difference in experience between someone who has seen your condition once or twice a month and a doctor who treats *only* your condition, day in and day out. Note that if you have a truly rare condition, even a specialist or subspecialist may have not seen it often.

5. *"Will you give me a photocopy of my lab results (or pathologist's report or radiology record) for my files?"*

First of all, you need these reports for your own medical record whether or not you decide to get additional opinions. (See chapter 6.)

Second, the information in these documents belongs to you, although many people believe they must get special permission to acquire it. Recent patient privacy legislation is clear on this point. Although you may be asked to pay a modest fee for photo-copying, you need no permission to obtain it. (See appendix E for information about privacy rules.) You also "own" your x–rays and have the right to request a set of them.

Third, because most doctors prefer not to spend time on pa-perwork, you may increase the probability that you get it quickly if you ask the receptionist or nurse for it. You don't really need to ask the physician to ask the office staff; you can approach them directly.

These questions will give you an opportunity to gather basic information about your condition. If this is a new doctor for you, it will give you an opportunity to see how well your personality style fits with his. And you can assess your confidence in this doctor's expertise.

When you talk to your doctor about your *treatment* ask these questions:

1. *"What other treatment options are available?"*

The speed of innovation in the treatment of some diseases is ex-traordinary.

- Evidence about the most effective treatments is summa-rized and released regularly but the doctor you are seeing may not have kept up with it.

- Scientists who conduct research studies to test new treat-ments are always seeking participants. Such studies are called clinical trials. See appendix D for a description and information about participating in one.

- The option of watchful waiting should always be consid-ered. "Watchful waiting" means carefully monitoring your condition over time to see if and how quickly the disease is progressing. It may progress so slowly that no treatment is required immediately.

You want to know about the full range of realistic options, and different physicians may know about different options or may view your options differently. You may decide to seek additional opinions to be confident that you are considering all the options available to you.

2. *"What are the pros and cons of the recommended treatment as opposed to other procedures, including watchful waiting?"*

While the doctor will recommend a specific treatment approach for you, there may be factors in your background or among your preferences that would lead to a different choice. All doctors are busy and can forget details in your history. A new doctor may not have noted, for example, that you had your spleen removed when you were twelve.

Ask your doctor to describe the thinking behind your treatment recommendation. Because there are substantial variations in treatment, it may be that one doctor will weigh the trade-offs for you in one way, whereas another will see them in another way.

3. *"How urgent is it that I begin treatment immediately?"*

You need to know the time course you are working with for a number of reasons.

- You need to plan how to fulfill your responsibilities and reorganize your immediate future to take care of yourself.

- If you are leaning toward getting at least one additional opinion, you need to know how fast you need to spring into action and how aggressive you need to be in getting this done.

4. *"What are the expected effects of different treatments?"*

You want to know about the most likely complications of this treatment as well as the less likely ones, and you want to know what are probable side effects as well as the rare side effects.

You want to know about short- and long-term changes—

mental and physical—that you can expect. You also want to know about the expected effects on your ability to work and do simple things like drive and read.

You may have choices among treatments and you need this kind of information to help you make them. Again, patients experience a range of side effects and tell their doctors about only some of them, so what you hear about a treatment from one physician may differ from what you hear from another.

Patient advocate Andrew Robinson notes that some physicians don't like to talk about side effects and complications because they think this information will make patients reluctant to proceed with treatment. "You may need to reassure your doctor that you know there are side effects and you want to be prepared for them."

5. "What will we do if this treatment is not successful?"

No treatment is effective 100 percent of the time. You want to know what your back-up treatment is. Not only will knowing this help you weigh your current choices, but knowledge that there is something else to try will help you weather the storm of despair so many of us feel between the time when we find out that our first treatment choice isn't working and our next doctor's appointment.

When you talk to your doctor about your *prognosis*, ask these questions:

1. "What is the prognosis for this condition in a person of my age and sex with my health history?"

This is a hard question to ask and the answer can be hard to listen to. The answer will be couched as a probability, since there is no certainty about this. The reason to ask it, however, is that it will help you think about the answer to the next question:

2. "How will the recommended treatment influence this prognosis?"

In coming up with your treatment plan, you will want to weigh the impact of the treatment on the quality of life with the probability that it will extend your life. A long, painful course of aggressive chemotherapy that will leave a person an invalid but extend life only slightly may be the right thing for some people but not for others.

Getting an answer that you don't like to the first question may be reason enough for you to seek another opinion.

But exploring the second question thoroughly with more than one physician is a pretty good idea especially if the proposed treatment is going to significantly change your life, permanently curtail your ability to function, visit considerable suffering, or financially damage your family.

How Do I Tell My Doctor I Want to Get Another Opinion?

Not only is there conventional wisdom about when to seek additional opinions about your diagnosis or treatment, but conventional wisdom also holds that any physician who is reluctant to help you get another opinion is not someone you should trust anyway.

Those words are easy to say, but actually talking to your physician about doing so can be difficult. Here are four approaches you can use to tell your doctor that you plan to seek an additional opinion:

1. "You know, this is a big decision for me and I would like to talk with another expert or two so that I feel completely confident in our treatment plan."

2. "You have been very helpful in explaining my diagnosis and possible treatment. I am interested in making sure I consider all my options before I move forward and am going to talk with some other specialists."

3. "My family insists that I get the opinions of a number of specialists before we move ahead," then: "I will schedule my next appointment and will be in touch."

4. If you are not asking for a referral for another opinion, you may choose not to tell your physician you are seeking another opinion.

But in all cases, schedule the next appointment before leaving the office. If you cannot arrange to get at least one additional opinion before then, reschedule it. Should you elect to be treated by the consulting physician, cancel this appointment. If you decide to be treated elsewhere, call the office and tell the receptionist or send a note to your physician and tell him so.

How Do I Actually Go about Getting Additional Opinions?

HOW MUCH DO I HAVE TO BE INVOLVED?
It is relatively rare to delegate the entire process of seeking additional opinions to someone else unless you are too ill to do it yourself. But some people are too overwhelmed to do the administrative work required to actually find the right doctors and set up the appointments. Some simply cannot bear to think about it.

Regardless of where you stand, you may want to ask a family member or close friend to share in some part of this task. That person can search the Web and seek out recommendations for expert opinions, arrange to have records delivered, and in some cases, arrange to get an opinion rendered without the patient actually showing up. (Note: you probably will be charged for the physician's time even if you are not physically present.)

> I simply did not want to deal with any of this. My husband and a close friend who is a doctor talked all the time. I was not interested in being included. They just told me when I had to show up. I knew that if I talked to my doctor, she would have told me everything but I didn't want to know. So my husband and his friend did all the talking for me. Only when I signed the consent form for surgery did I see the words "renal cell carcinoma"—and realize or admit to myself—that it was cancer.
>
> Nina, 36—professor

WHICH DOCTOR?
If your diagnosing physician did not make a referral to another specialist at your request, a trusted internist, family physician, or nurse practitioner may be a good source of recommendations. In addition, you will want to talk to everyone you know and have

them talk to everyone they know to get the names of doctors and hospitals that have expertise in treating your disease.

Many physicians and nurses I talked to recommended getting additional opinions outside of the hospital with which your first hospital was affiliated, on the grounds that doctors in a hospital will tend to be in agreement. The need for collegiality may bias the opinion in unexpected ways. In addition, protocols for treating a given condition vary among hospitals and you want to know your full range of treatment options.

If you live in a small community, look in a larger city for a physician to give you a consultation, if possible. This will alleviate any social pressures that may influence doctors' deference to one another's expertise, which has been documented to take place in small medical communities.

When selecting a physician, think about your concerns. For certain, you are looking for a physician who treats your disease specifically. But you may want advice from a different type of specialist. For example, if your first doctor is a surgeon and wants to take your gall bladder out because you have had abdominal pain, you may want to go to a gastroenterologist (an internal medicine specialist with training about organs in the abdomen) who might first try a nonsurgical approach.

Seeking an opinion from a physician at an academic medical center makes sense, since (a) there is a greater likelihood that you will find a specialist who has treated people with your condition frequently, and (b) faculty generally are required to participate in research and so are more likely to be aware of the latest evidence reviews that summarize what is known about the treatments available to you, as well as the clinical trials that might offer you additional choices.

Most medical centers, academic or otherwise, have referral services that can match you with a physician who is a specialist in your condition.

See chapter 4 for a detailed description of how to find doctors and check their credentials.

DOES INSURANCE COVER THIS?
Talk with your insurance company or managed care plan about coverage for additional opinions. See chapter 8 for more

suggestions about making good use of your health plan or insurance.

Some states, including New York and California, mandate coverage of second surgical opinions, and many health plans cover them without the mandate. There are also different ways of getting additional opinions. Medicare will not pay for a second opinion unless the patient comes to the office, whereas other plans will pay for a second physician to review the paperwork and test results. Some health plans require that you make a request for coverage of another opinion before you seek one. This is to discourage people from "doctor shopping"—going from doctor to doctor until they find one who will do what they want them to.

The Web has sparked a whole new industry of "second opinion factories," some of which are affiliated with academic medical centers and others with freestanding entrepreneurial ventures. Some of these services are portals to reputable specialty services for uncommon conditions at academic medical centers, i.e., they provide contact information so that you can call to get an appointment. Others just offer to take a look at your tests and provide an opinion about the diagnosis or treatment. Use caution and ask questions when considering such services.

Do not ask for an additional opinion without arranging to pay for it.

WHAT DO I TELL THE CONSULTING PHYSICIAN'S OFFICE STAFF?

When you call, tell the receptionist that you are seeking an opinion about your specific diagnosis or treatment. Identify who your original physician is and the referral source, even though you may have been referred by the hospital's referral service, a colleague, or family member. Also note what your question is and mention its urgency. "I was diagnosed with X on Monday. My doctor recommended that I have surgery within the month and I want to be certain this is the only treatment available to me."

Chapter 6 describes how to work with office staff to make good use of your time with the physician.

WHAT SHOULD I EXPECT OF THE OPINION?

The consulting physician will talk with you about your health history, examine you, and review your records. She will prepare a written report that will be sent to you and to your first doctor. He or she may call your diagnosing physician with your permission, especially if there is a big difference in their views and if there is time urgency.

It may be that you will get a complete confirmation of what your first physician told you about the diagnosis and treatment. If so, the question becomes who do you want to treat you? This is an especially important question *if* the reason you sought an additional opinion was that you didn't really have confidence in your first physician and he or she was proposing to treat you or to coordinate your care.

However, it may also be the case that the physician offering the opinion has a very different view of the situation, whether it is about the diagnosis, the treatment, its urgency, or the prognosis. Remember, all diagnoses and recommendations are probability statements, and often there are several reasonable alternatives.

If you have confidence in your diagnosing doctor, after you have gotten additional opinions about your diagnosis and/or possible courses of action, you will want to bring this information back to your original doctor to discuss what you have found.

How Do I Make Sense of What I Learn?

The aim of seeking additional opinions is to have confidence that you are going to receive the treatment for your condition that is best for you, one that meets your needs and preferences and will give you the best possible outcome. Regardless of whether you seek additional opinions, the final decision about your treatment and the doctors who will deliver it will be powerfully influenced by the kind of person you are and the life you are leading.

Some of the considerations you will bring to bear on this decision are completely practical: Gara, fifty-three, an athletic facility manager, said, "I need to be able to drive for my job and the treatment that was going to keep me off the road for six months was out of the question."

Some of them will have to do with your preferences. Juan,

seventy-eight, a media consultant, said, "I hate—can I tell you, *hate* to throw up. That really affected my treatment choice in the end." And some of them have to do with your values:

> I want to be as engaged with my family and friends and stay as active as I can for as long as I can. I don't want to chance a long fading illness because of treatment that maybe *maybe* will give me another couple months. I don't want my babies to remember me that way.
>
> Suzanne, 36—economist

The information you have gathered about your condition and your options is only a part of what goes into your plan for how to respond to this devastating diagnosis. Chapter 10 talks about how to blend expert opinion with your own needs when you have choices among treatment plans.

Get Timely Care

Your aim is to confirm your diagnosis, consult with physicians, and make decisions about treatment in a timely manner.

I made forty-seven phone calls to a myriad of different sources to secure my first appointment with the doctor I wanted to see. I remember
telephoning my minister to express my exhaustion and my inability to
access the institutions and doctors I needed. It was so difficult. I was
surprised at my lack of ease in networking myself into this excellent institution and I thought to myself, "Everyone with cancer wants to live
and now I, too, am in a line searching and asking to be included in the
need to live." I was aghast at this epiphany.

Maral, 44—writer

CALLING FOR AN APPOINTMENT to see a new specialist,
scheduling a test, getting your records to the office ahead of
time, and making sure the specialist calls your doctor or that the
test results are sent to the right person—these small tasks can
seem daunting when you are worried and upset and are not sure
which of these you have to do for yourself.

Even if your diagnosis gives you some breathing room and
your appointments don't have to be scheduled immediately, they
should be done in a couple weeks. Some people procrastinate about
following up on referrals or finding new doctors. They hesitate because finding out more may confirm how serious their diagnosis really is. Others put it off because they are intimidated by the prospect
of trying to convince a highly regarded busy specialist to make an
exception and see them soon. Yet others just breeze through this
process as if they were making an appointment for a haircut.

Regardless of how you and your loved ones approach getting consultations and tests quickly, this chapter provides some
principles and pieces of information that will help smooth your

way. It starts with a few facts you need to know about how health care for serious illness is generally organized; this will reduce some of the surprises you might encounter. Then it discusses what staff and physicians say about urgent consultations and taking on new patients.

Most of the physicians and nurses I spoke with recommended taking a partner with you to your appointments, and this chapter gives you some information on who that partner should be and what he or she can do to help you.

Who collects and manages all the information that you are generating? Often you or your partner does. This chapter also discusses the ins and outs of how you can make sure the right information about you gets to the right place at the right time, to avoid unnecessary delays, and you'll hear about the "kit" you will want to take with you to each appointment.

There is a section for people who struggle when making appointments, who are uncertain how to convey the urgency they feel, and are uncomfortable asking for what they need. Tips on what you should say and how the scheduler might respond are included here.

And finally, it is important for you to know a little about privacy and also about informed consent, two topics that you are going to address (with your signature, if not your attention) frequently over the coming weeks. They are both big deals for doctors, nurses, and hospitals these days. While you probably feel that you would be willing to sign almost anything to get your condition under control, it's a good idea to have a general understanding of what these topics mean in the medical world.

A Few Facts You Should Know

Specialists see people on an urgent basis all the time. Most of them are organized to do so. Specialists who treat serious diseases are always asked to see people sooner rather than later. Don't feel you are being pushy or asking a favor by requesting an urgent appointment. You need to be very clear when you call about the urgency of your situation, but you should expect that any doctor you call with this request will want to make his or her own determination of how quickly you need to be seen.

"There is a medical and a humanistic answer to who needs to be seen immediately: With acute leukemia, for example, patients need to be seen the same day; that's medical. Otherwise, unless there is a medical reason to see them sooner, we try to get *all* patients in within five days because we know how hard it is for them. Waiting is not humanistic. We try to give scan results the same day too, for the same reason," said Larry Shulman, an oncologist at Dana Farber Cancer Center in Boston.

You may need to have the relevant information ready to fax upon request. (See "The Right Information..." page 115.) And you will definitely need to rearrange your schedule to accommodate your doctor's.

Most physicians honor urgent requests from other physicians and nurses. Ask your physician or nurse practitioner to make a referral; this increases the chance that you will get an appointment with an in-demand specialist. People run into trouble with this when they are seeking additional opinions without support from the physician who diagnosed their condition (see chapter 5). If this is the case, consider asking your primary care provider to refer you to physicians you have independently identified.

Some specialists—especially very well-known ones—have full practices and may not be taking new patients within the window of time in which you need to be seen. They may, however, be willing to see you for a one-time consultation to confirm your diagnosis or weigh in on your proposed treatment plan. If you are determined to be treated by this person, you might ask the referring doctor or your regular doctor to intervene. (See "Making Appointments—What Do You Say?" page 107.)

Many specialists take only selected insurance or none. Depending on your financial circumstances and the cost of the anticipated procedures, it will be very important to ask whether the doctor takes your insurance when calling to see if you can get an appointment. (See page 108, and chapter 8 on paying for care.)

Don't throw away paper. There are three kinds of paper you have to keep track of during this time:

- Any new information that you generate: test and lab results; and your own notes about what doctors you have seen, what you have learned, and the informed consent forms you have signed, even if you did not read them at the time

- Prescriptions for medications (and any receipts) and referrals for tests

- All the papers that involve payment for services. If you can't deal with the latter right now, get a shoe box and dump them in there. This will not be a good permanent solution, but it'll do for the first few weeks.

The former—all the test results that led to your diagnosis, all the informed consent forms, all prescriptions and test orders—you need to hang onto copies of those as if your life depends on it. It may.

Note that, if you are part of an integrated health system with an electronic medical record, all this information may be stored in that record. In that case, the paper records are important if you are seen by a physician outside your system. The majority of Americans still do not have access to electronic medical records. If you do—or think you do—you may want to check to be sure and to confirm what information is in your record and which physicians can obtain access to it.

Professional advice about health-care-related finances and insurance is available. Gaps in the organization of American health care have sparked the development of a variety of "specialist" services that can help with some of the tasks of getting the care you need. These services will advise you about which specialists you may want to see and treatments you may want to pursue, make referrals to your choices, and help coordinate your care. Most, though not all of them, cost money. None of them will work magic and none of them do everything. All of them require a careful check before you make a commitment. Appendix G describes a number of different kinds of services that have sprung up and gives you ideas about how to find them.

What Scheduling Staff and Physicians Say about Urgent Consultations and Taking on New Patients

"The best way to do this is to have the referring physician make the appointment or ask your primary care provider to do it," said the manager of a multidisciplinary clinic in New Mexico. "Most likely they'll call and talk to the doctor and then you call later and talk to the scheduler."

A physician executive in a health plan in Iowa, said, "People often ask their doctors which treatment approach they would recommend for their own wife or child. I think it's just as reasonable to ask 'if one of your family members was making this decision, how much time would you say they had to make it?' Physicians don't automatically give this information, but I think people need to know objectively how much of a medical crisis this is."

The practice manager of a busy surgical practice in Oregon, said, "People don't understand that once they have been diagnosed, they can't just have surgery the next day unless it is a stroke or heart attack—really an emergency. Usually you have to come off all the drugs you are taking, talk with the anesthesiologist, and get preauthorization from your insurance company."

"Make friends with nurses, office staff, and schedulers. Get to know them on a first-name basis. They are the ones who control access to the physician and to your own information. It's better to have them on your team," said a cardiology practice manager in New York City. "But if you appear to be sucking up or give the impression that you think you are more worthy than other patients who are also seriously ill, it may be counterproductive," added a nephrologist in private practice in Arkansas. "Be polite, be courteous, be persistently pleasant, but don't ask them to go bowling with you."

The manager of a large oncology practice in Georgia, said, "Getting consult notes from each doctor is important. You usually can't get them at the end of your appointment. Unless your doctor belongs to a practice that uses computers to share medical records, you will probably have to wait at least seventy-two hours until your doctor dictates her notes and they are typed and sent back to her office."

"It's best that someone call who is not going to break down if I say 'the next opening is in two weeks,'" said a scheduler and receptionist in an oncology practice in Oregon. "One thing that works is to let the scheduler know that you would like to be on the cancellation list."

Making Appointments: What Do You Say?

Whether or not you are struggling to get yourself to schedule an appointment with a specialist to confirm your diagnosis or to talk about treatment options, you may want to read through this script before you pick up the phone.

If you were referred to this new doctor by another physician, the referring physician may call in advance to ask the new doctor to see you. If you have trouble getting an appointment, you may wish to ask the referring doctor to intercede or recommend another specialist.

Regardless of whether your physician has called ahead, you will also be calling to ask the receptionist of a busy professional to see you as soon as possible. If you feel uncertain, use these words and considerations as a guide.

"Hello, this is ___. I would like to make an appointment to see Dr. X. Are you the right person to talk to?" In many practices and specialty treatment centers, the person who answers the phone is not the scheduler.

"I was diagnosed last Wednesday with ___." Be as specific as you can about your diagnosis—mention the formal name of the disease and what you know about how advanced it is.

"I was referred by ___." If you were referred by your own physician or a specialist you saw recently, this is the name to use. If you learned about this physician from a former patient or the hospital referral service, or found the name on the Internet or in a reference book, mention this.

"I would like to see Dr. X for ___." Say what it is that you are seeking. An opinion about your original diagnosis? An opinion about your treatment options? An opinion from a different specialty about your situation altogether? To talk about receiving ongoing care from this physician?

"Dr. Z [the physician who made the initial diagnosis] said that this is urgent—that I must get this taken care of right away—so I would like an appointment as soon as possible. Can you tell me when that might be?" There are a few things to think about here:

How urgent *is* this? Is your disease progressing so quickly that you may die if you do not have this consultation immediately? If so, the doctor who referred you to the specialist should have already called or told you exactly what to say. Or is the urgency you feel the result of the uncertainty about your body and about your future? Both are legitimate reasons to want an appointment right away—tomorrow, for example. Experienced schedulers and practice managers know that one or both motivations may be operating. But your idea of "right away" may not work for this doctor, and you should be prepared for this. How long can you wait and not drive yourself nuts with anxiety?

Alternatively, next year might be too soon for those of us who would prefer not to know much more about our disease. You and your loved ones need to watch that you don't allow the lack of availability of an appointment with a specific physician serve as an excuse to do nothing.

Ask yourself whether seeing this particular doctor is so important to you that, despite your worry, you can wait until the week after next or until next month for an appointment—or do you just need to be seen very soon by any really good doctor who can help figure out your situation?

"I have Y insurance coverage. Does Dr. X participate in this plan? And if not, how much does a consultation cost?" Consultations with specialists are almost always expensive, which is not a reason not to see them but is a reason to ask. You have had enough surprises and this is one you can avoid.

You may have chosen to see a particular specialist because she is the best one to treat your condition who takes your insurance and who practices near you, in which case you are on safe ground here. But if you got this referral from another doctor or through your own research, you will want to ask about payment. You should not assume that a physician who accepts your insurance will necessarily refer you only to other doctors who also take it. Choosing a physician to treat you over the long term who does not participate in your insurance plan can be very expensive. (See chapter 8 for ideas about how to approach this decision.)

Here are some answers you may get and ideas about how to respond:

"Sure. Can you come in next Tuesday at two o'clock and can you please send your file immediately?" Good. Ask for the fax number, then go home or to the copy shop and fax your medical record to them, along with a cover sheet confirming the date and time of your appointment, and your contact information. Fax only critical information about the current problem, for example, the referring doctor's note, a biopsy, or critical lab results that help define the problem. See "The Right Information about You..., page 115," for guidance about who to include.

"Dr. X isn't taking any new patients right now." Mention that you want to see this specialist because of his or her outstanding reputation for treating similar cases, which is surely true. Alternatively, beseeching and crying sometimes work. Practice managers, schedulers, and physicians I talked to noted that there is a big difference between taking on a new complicated case and a one-time appointment to confirm a diagnosis or discuss a treatment plan. Besides, until you meet this new doctor, you aren't sure yourself that you want anything more than that from her. So it may help your chances to reiterate that you are only looking for a consultation. If you succeed and you meet the physician and you feel this is someone you really would like to work with for your treatment, you can raise the issue in person, rather than with the scheduler or practice manager.

"Dr. X's earliest opening is three months from now." You can see if the three-month timeframe is flexible if you just want a consultation. Or you can ask if Dr. X will refer you to a colleague.

This is slightly chancy—you don't know Dr. X, don't know whether you trust his judgment and he certainly doesn't know your case—but if you have heard really good things about him from a number of independent sources, it may be worthwhile to give it a try. You may want to scout around about the doctor he refers you to before you proceed, however. In large physician groups, this kind of referral may land you with the newest doctor in the practice or the one with the most openings on her schedule.

Many specialists I interviewed do not turn away patients. They look at the information about the diagnosis, make a determination about the urgency and if they are unable to take on a complicated and urgent case right then, they make a referral to someone they have confidence will be able to provide good care, based on the specifics of the case.

In an emergency, I was once passed off from one senior physician to another in the middle of a diagnosis because the first one had a skiing vacation planned. I was not that familiar with the first guy but trusted that he wouldn't just refer me to any old physician, given that he had seen me once and knew that I was very sick and needed someone who could treat this fast-moving disease.

Taking along a Partner

The role of "partner" is one that is, for many, unique to this time when you are going to try to find out information about your condition and may not be feeling very sick. A partner is the person who helps you do the things you must do during this time: make appointments, go to the doctor, have diagnostic tests done, collect test results, and chart notes. This person may or may not be the one to help you think through your options for treatment, work, and managing your responsibilities in the future. This depends on your relationship and your preferences.

A partner is your advocate; that is, he or she is on your side and acts in your interests at your request. This may mean that the person will take on a *dominant* role, as a taxi driver did for his aging mother; an *equal* role, as my husband did for me; or a *helping* role, as one single woman's friends did for her. But whatever the role, it must be according to your wishes.

This is your life. This is your diagnosis. This disease or condition is taking place in your body. You are the one who will make the final decision about your course of action. You are the one who will undergo the treatment and live with its effects. And you are the one to determine who accompanies you on this initial technical part of the journey and how they can be most helpful to you. (See "Putting Out the Fire," page 58.)

The one thing that everyone I talked to agreed upon, whether they were the person with the diagnosis, their family or friends, doctors, nurses, or clergy, is that it is important to take someone else with you when you go to your doctors' appointments. The partner role can be far larger and more involved than just going to medical appointments, but it is one of the few roles that cut across all conditions, all ages, and all levels of medical sophistication.

WHY TAKE SOMEONE WITH YOU TO YOUR APPOINTMENTS?

One young woman with a large extended family always took a family member—husband, aunt, brother-in-law, distant cousin—to her appointments, prompting her physician to comment that he now could fill in the entire family tree.

Hannah, thirty-seven, a single parent, described how she "maintained a companions' notebook—I asked that whoever accompanied me that day take notes about what the doctors said, what I asked, and what the doctor's answers were. It helped me keep all the information in order and in one place. It also helped me keep track of which questions I already asked."

Meryl, fifty-seven, a college president, took her daughter and her husband to all appointments: "Each of us had such different perspectives and asked different questions!"

Harry, seventy-eight, a retired advertising executive, who always accompanied his daughter to appointments said, "Even if there are three of us [family members] in the room, we each remember different things that were said—and sometimes the things we remember have different meanings to us and we have to sort them out—and sometimes get clarification from the doctor."

There are four main reasons to take someone with you to medical appointments. First, it is difficult to absorb all the unfamiliar technical information that is discussed and which may be important to weigh as you make decisions. A partner can make a record of what is said so you can revisit it later, figure out if you understand it, and plan how to ask the doctor to explain something further or add to what you already know.

Second, your distress about your diagnosis and the meaning of this information about your future can affect your ability to listen and understand. A partner can help you remember important considerations you may have forgotten or can remind you of your intentions. For example, your sister can remind you that you didn't want to make a decision about treatment during the appointment and can ask the doctor for some time to think about it.

Third, it may be hard to question, disagree, or advocate for your own best interests when you feel that your doctor holds your life in her hands. A partner can take on those tasks, can ask for clarification, and can ask hard questions for you.

And finally, you may be able to distract yourself from the stark facts of your condition some of the time, but it is difficult to do this when you are talking to your doctor. Or you may be dwelling on the worst-case scenario. In either case, having someone else hear the words your doctor says and write them down to read later can steady you and help you feel less isolated in your knowledge about what is going on.

A JOB DESCRIPTION FOR YOUR PARTNER

Because having a partner with you during doctor visits is so important and because *being* such a partner is more than just a chore, you may wish to share the following list of dos and don'ts with your partner or potential partners.

If you are a partner, you *will*:

- Agree to attend the appointment, freeing at least two hours *past* the time the appointment should end in case of delays.

- Twenty-four hours ahead of time, confirm to the diagnosed person that you will be there. Go over arrangements about transportation, address of facility, telephone number, and time.

- Ask the diagnosed person what role you should play. For example:

  — Should I sit quietly and take notes or do you want me to participate? If so, how?

— Should I ask questions if something is not clear to *me?*

— Are there questions you would like me to ask so you don't have to?

— Is there anything you can think of that I should absolutely say or not say?

- Arrive at the assigned place fifteen minutes ahead of time with paper and pen.

- Do as the diagnosed person has requested during the appointment.

- Afterward, discuss what happened during the appointment according to the wishes of the diagnosed person.

- Provide a readable version of notes taken during the appointment that day or the next.

As a partner, you *will not:*

- Talk with others about what happened during the appointment or express opinions about the diagnosed person's decisions without explicit permission, even with family members. It is important that you and the diagnosed person discuss this.

- Forget the appointment or be late. Doing so can have untold meaning to the diagnosed person. Although under ordinary circumstances such lapses can be seen as casual lateness or simple carelessness, for someone who is has a life–threatening condition, not appearing at the designated time can be a betrayal of trust. It can cause panic and avoidable emotional pain, as well as cause an important appointment to be missed.

- Take on this responsibility if you are unable or unwilling to fulfill it fully.

The extent to which the person who accompanies you to doctors' appointments has an ongoing role outside of going to appointments depends on your circumstances and preferences.

I talked to people whose families were unwilling to do much more. One seventy-year-old executive described how his adult children kept telling him he "would be fine, just fine," and were unavailable to come to appointments while his wife, who came to most doctors' appointments, excused herself from talking about what they had learned, telling him that he needed to make the treatment decisions himself, since he had to live with the consequences.

Some people choose to limit the role of their partners to note-taking.

> I have educated myself and am far more sophisticated about my treatment choices than anyone I might bring to appointments. Plus I feel like I have a good relationship with a number of specialists and can call them for advice. I've pretty much decided to do this alone.
>
> Sharon, 57—university dean

If you are in the hospital and are feeling that you may not be thinking clearly, you may want to choose one family member to serve as the spokesperson for you with the doctors and hospital staff. Make sure that the spokesperson is someone who you trust and who understands your wishes.

During a long stay in an intensive care unit when I was twenty, my mother had to repeatedly explain to the doctors that they had to talk to *me* about what was going on, not her. If I didn't feel like I could make a decision about my care—if it was too complicated or scary, I would tell her and she would make it.

At the hospital, ask your family to organize themselves so that someone is always there with you, if possible. "If your mom were your five-year-old daughter, you would be here all the time. You have to be there for her. There isn't enough nursing care to really care for people—they are stretched too thin," commented internist/medical journalist Teresa Schrader.

The Right Information about You at the
Right Place at the Right Time

"A critical trigger is that all the paperwork is together. For example, if a doctor doesn't have your most recent MRI or your medical history, she can't schedule surgery. The last thing you want to hear is, 'I'll get back to you when your pathology report arrives,'" said Ann Seger, a practice manager in Eugene, Oregon.

You are undoubtedly generating a lot of new information that every physician you see is going to need. Why can't you just ask for your doctors to send it to the right people?

You can. And they will. Perhaps not in time for your appointment with another doctor. Or perhaps not *all* the test results, meaning you have to repeat a test. Don't take a chance on this. No one is more concerned that you get the best care than you are, so take it upon yourself to get and keep these records. The information in your medical record—test results, lab reports, and notes—is yours, and legally, you must be able to get copies within thirty days. (You may be asked to pay for photocopying.)

But thirty days is a long time to wait when you are trying to settle on what you are going to do about this diagnosis. So here's what you do: you tell the doctor and the nurse and the office staff that you need the test results and the notes for another appointment—say when that is—and ask when is the soonest you could possibly get a copy of them. Tell them that you will come back and pick them up. Could they photocopy them now? When can you stop by to get them?

And then call before you come to pick them up, to make sure they are ready.

If you are receiving all your care within an HMO or health-care system with a shared electronic medical record, you will not need to do this as long as all your physicians have access to your record. If, however, you go outside your system or, like most of us, you receive your care from doctors who have no formal affiliation with one another—even if they work one floor away from one another in an office building—you will be better off if you take charge of this new information and add it to the medical chart you carry with you.

Beware of handing over too much of a good thing, however. Your new specialist probably doesn't need your school immunization records or the prescription you once had for reading glasses. Neat, organized, and to the point is what we are working toward here.

Geriatrician James Cooper said, "I have been assaulted by earnest patients with two-hundred-page medical records that are so overpowering in size and complexity that they are hard to read. Information overload obscures important items—and I don't get reimbursed for reading your history, even if you send it ahead of time."

Here are the ingredients of the record that any physician will want to see before he examines you:

- Notes and laboratory results related to the problem at hand, starting when you first noticed a symptom/sign of the illness

- Active medical problems. This means problems for which you receive treatment periodically. Make a list of recurring problems you have had since adulthood and indicate the year last treated. The physician can scan the list and ask for more information if needed.

- Allergies. Don't forget to include allergies to nickel or latex.

- All current medication, including prescription and over-the-counter drugs, their exact doses and frequencies

- If surgery is contemplated, all medications in the last year (looking particularly for steroids)

- Any serious illness or hospitalizations in the past two years

- Any problems *ever* from surgery (excess bleeding, anesthesia sensitivity)

- Anything any physician or nurse ever told you to "be sure to tell your doctors"

Other than the notes about your current serious problem, all this information should fit on one page, two at the most. You don't need to write long explanations—your doctor will ask you about the items that need elaboration. Note that you will undoubtedly be asked to fill out a registration form that may include some of this information for the clinic's records.

YOUR PERSONAL HEALTH KIT

As long as we are talking about how to prepare for getting timely care, let me make one somewhat idiosyncratic suggestion based on far too much experience in waiting rooms: You need luggage.

Okay, not like a suitcase or anything. Rather, you need a particular kind of bag that accompanies you everywhere on your journey as you pass the hours in waiting rooms and examining rooms.

It should be a sturdy bag—even a grocery or shopping bag with handles will do. Staple a card with your name, address, and cell and home telephone numbers to the inside.

Before you leave the house for any medical appointments, check to make sure these things are in it:

- A notebook that contains

  — Your health insurance number and the telephone numbers for your plan

  — All your physicians' and hospital names, addresses and telephone numbers, the names of the nurses and the office staff

  — Chronological notes from physician visits

- Your medical record file as described above

- A manila envelope for all paper related to insurance and payment of medical expenses

- Personal telephone number list

- A portable charger for your mobile phone

- A book, a magazine, a puzzle, or your knitting

- A snack and a bottle of water

You are going to spend unpredictable amounts of time waiting in medical offices. You need the mobile phone and charger because you can't afford to be out of touch if you are trying to coordinate appointments. You don't want to be isolated from friends and family. And since you are easily distractible right now, you may lose stuff. Keep everything in the bag.

This is the voice of experience talking. Give it a try.

Now Is the Time to Learn a Little about Privacy and Informed Consent

"No, it's not," you say. "I don't care who knows what about me as long as I get this taken care of."

Not so fast.

Privacy in health care has many meanings. Understanding these meanings can influence the quality of your care and your ability to maintain your dignity and independence while you are ill and in treatment. And it may affect your long-term employability and insurability.

Plus, you don't actually have to *do* anything about privacy right now. You just have to *know* about it so that you can consider it in your choice of doctors and can exercise your options whenever you choose.

On the other hand, you may already have some concern about who knows your diagnosis and what it might mean if, for example, your employer found out about it. If you are worried and don't know how to proceed, this section will orient you to the topic and point you toward more specific help.

Being able to trust your doctors and share with them everything they need to know is a critical part of what you do to get the best and right health care. But some people don't do this; they omit pieces of their medical history, they ask their doctors or nurses not to record the results of a test, or they pay out of pocket because they think—in some cases rightly so—that health information will be shared with an employer or insurer and that this, in turn, will result in the loss of work or insurance.

You are no doubt familiar with the idea that when you talk to your doctor, you are protected by doctor–patient confidentiality— you may associate this with the Hippocratic Oath that all physicians take upon graduation from medical school in which they pledge to "keep secret" what they know about you. Many of us assume that there are protections similar to lawyer–client privilege operating in our relationship with our doctors.

It may surprise you to learn that until recently, doctor–patient confidentiality was an ethical standard and that it was not legally enforceable. It was a standard that physicians found increasingly difficult to uphold. There are now laws and contracts that supersede that standard, and the confidentiality of your records is thus dependent on a mix of your condition or disease, your doctor, the institution, and your own choices. For example, doctors sign contracts with hospitals and health plans about the kind of information they will provide on patients. This means that some information about you is going to be shared without your explicit permission.

While most of us have long made assumptions about our privacy as patients, until recently there was really nothing protecting information about our health from public eyes except this ethical standard, plus an inconsistent smattering of local and state regulations.

As medicine and communications technology became more sophisticated, this disorganized approach hurt people: someone's genetic disorder is revealed to her employer through careless record-keeping and she loses her job; hundreds of people's medical histories, social security numbers, and job status are mistakenly posted on the Internet for months, leading to a widespread identity theft.

Protections were needed.

In 2003, rules that require doctors and insurance companies to protect patients' privacy came into effect, as required by Congress in the 1996 Health Insurance Portability and Accountability

Act (HIPAA). These rules don't take care of every instance but do put in place two provisions important for you: that you have a legal right to get a copy of your medical record, and that your doctor and the insurance company or health plan is not allowed to share information about you with your employer.

Why, you may ask, would I care who saw my health information? Well, would you make any of these statements about yourself?

- My business will suffer because people will think I can't deliver.

- Employers will be worried about hiring me—why should they invest in someone who they think they can't depend upon?

- I don't want my friends and colleagues to see me as weak or sick.

- My daughter might not be able to get a job if it is known that I have an inheritable condition.

- I have an incurable disease that is progressive and I don't want anyone else to know about it until they have to.

- It ain't nobody's business but my own.

If you would not make these statements, you still should know that you are not required to tell your employer what your diagnosis is in order to be protected under the Family and Medical Leave Act (FMLA) (see chapter 7 for more information) and that you will be asked throughout your encounters with the health-care system to sign forms related to information privacy. If you have read such a form carefully, you know that usually it describes the institution's rights in making use of your personal information, and that signing it means that it has informed you that the institution has protections in place but that they will also share information about you when it deems it appropriate. (See appendix E for a description of the rights guaranteed to you as a patient and as an employee under HIPAA and a list of resources that provide further explanation of the law.)

However, if you *would* make any one of these statements, you need to know that for health-care treatment and the payment of claims, the law assumes that this information can be shared *without* your permission. There is a section of the law that says that you can request a restriction of the information, but the doctor must agree in order to make it binding.

So if you are concerned about either your health plan or your employer getting information about you—test results confirming your diagnosis, for example—tell your physician that you are concerned about keeping this information private. Although a doctor is *allowed* to do this, this doctor and her office staff are not *required* to. You must raise the issue and request that they assist you in restricting access to this information. Note also that employers are not covered by the HIPAA privacy rule, and so can collect information directly from employees, for example, from their preemployment screening, employee assistance, and wellness programs.

Janlori Goldman, one of the architects of HIPAA and director of the Privacy Project, says, "The whole issue of privacy in health care is so that people have some degree of dignity and control, so that they can make a choice whether or not to share information that makes them vulnerable. If it is important to you—for whatever reason—to be seen by your friends or at work as someone who doesn't have cancer or MS—it should be your decision, not one made for you by your doctor or some hospital administrator. At the most basic, this has to be negotiated with your doctor and you have to be able to trust that your concerns will be honored."

A final note: In the course of interviewing practice managers and hospital staff for this book, I found that they described some pretty strict interpretations of HIPAA, many of which set up barriers to patients trying to move their information quickly among various doctors and hospitals. When I asked them about how their policies compared to HIPAA itself, they were adamant: because they are nervous about liability, they sometimes go beyond what is required just to be safe. And, after all, enforcing the policies as they are interpreted in their institution is part of their job description.

This suggests that you can learn about your rights from the resources listed in appendix E, but if an institution's HIPAA policy seems to be contradicted by what you see there, this may not be the time to spend your energy picking a fight. If the interpretation is overly restrictive, you can point out that information can be shared if there is an urgent need. If the interpretation seems overly lax, you can file a complaint to the United States Department of Health and Human Services. The Health Privacy Project provides good instructions about how to do so: www.health privacy.org.

WHAT ARE ALL THESE INFORMED CONSENT FORMS FOR?

I always thought informed consent was a quirk of the medical care system—you know, doctors and hospitals protecting themselves from lawsuits. All of a sudden I was consenting to treatments that posed very real—and high—risks. I realize now that informed consent is for me, the patient. It has protected me from a doctor who wanted to try an experimental drug whose side effects would have forced me to quit my job.

Raphael, 38—designer

You no doubt have signed informed consent forms when you received your prescription drugs, or before you got medical tests, procedures, or operations in the past. So you are familiar with the idea that you must be told about the risks and possible side effects of the treatment you are going to receive.

When you have a life-altering condition or disease, informed consent takes on new significance. During this time, the tests you undergo may be more intrusive and thus more dangerous. And because your doctors' assessment and clear communication of your diagnosis and prognosis, treatment alternatives, and their possible side effects will powerfully influence your decisions about treatment, informed consent is the legal obligation of the doctor to make sure that you understand the reasoning behind a course of action—and the possible implications of it.

Consider, as you are asked to sign these forms, that informed consent is often not given in light of other preexisting conditions. For example, the risks of coronary bypass surgery described in an informed consent document are often for the general population, not relative to the personal circumstances of an individual patient who may have other conditions that increase her risk of complications.

"Informed consent frequently doesn't include the risks [of the procedure at a particular institution or] of the specific doctors performing surgery or delivering other care," said Charles Inlander, former president of the People's Medical Society. "And there is huge variation in outcomes based on each of these variables. We are also rarely given the risks of the nontreatment alternative, for example, what is the difference in my risks if I *do* get this treatment versus if I *don't* get it? When you buy a car, you get informed consent on a sticker on the window."

Others would point out that miles per gallon and test track stopping distance does not inform you of your risk of dying in that car. Neither do anticipated energy costs tell you how much you will pay in repair bills or how long that new refrigerator will last. More information is better than none, but it is likely that no document will ever give you all the information you would like.

Informed consent is required by law to include the following. The "informed" part of informed consent means that you have been told:

- *Your diagnosis.* Or at least what is known about your diagnosis to date.

- *The purpose of the test, procedure or treatment.* Your doctor must tell you what information the test will provide or how the treatment will affect the progression of your disease or condition.

- *What will happen during the test, procedure, or treatment.* Will you receive drugs intravenously or orally? Will you be sedated during the procedure? What exactly is going to happen to which body parts?

- *How this is expected to affect you.* What are the benefits and risks of the treatment or procedure in question? How long does it usually take to recover? How will it influence your ability to function in the short and long term? How long you are expected to be in the hospital? Will receiving this treatment limit your treatment options in the future?

- *What alternative options you may have, their possible benefits, and side effects.* What other drugs are available that might achieve the same outcome? Are there other tests that will find the same information? All options should be

described, regardless of their cost and regardless of
whether the treatment or test is covered by your
insurance.

- *The consequences of deciding not to go ahead with the test, procedure,
  or treatment or of waiting for a few months to decide.* If you ask a
  hard question, for example, "How long do people usually
  live with my stage of this disease?" your doctor must
  answer you truthfully.

Oncologist Karen Antman said, "I find that people sometimes ask
hard questions and don't really want to know the answer. I say 'If
you ask, I must tell you the truth. But if you don't want to hear
the answer you can ask for someone else—a family member, for
example—to hear the answer.'"

The "consent" part of informed consent means that you understand what has been said. You appreciate what is reasonably
expected to happen and whether or not you go ahead with this. It
means:

- *You are making this decision on your own free will.* Are you in
  terrible pain? Do you still have unanswered questions
  about the treatment and procedure and its risks? Are you
  under the influence of medication that clouds your judgment? If you answered yes to any of these questions, you
  may not be in any condition to give voluntary consent
  and should not sign it. It may be that because of your
  condition, your legally authorized representative will
  make these decisions. This is one reason it is a good idea
  to talk about your wishes with someone you trust to act
  on your wishes. (See chapter 8 for ideas about how to do
  this.)

  If your mind is clear enough for you to comprehend
  the information and you want to consent to the test or
  procedure, you can sign and date the informed consent
  documents. They will be put in your medical file and you
  should ask for your own signed copy for your records.

- *You can revoke your consent at any time.* If the treatment or surgery is scheduled for another day and you are unsure
  about what you have been told and want to think about
  it, sign the form and take it home. Call your doctor with

questions. If you decide to revoke your consent and cancel your treatment, you can do so—you are not bound by the form you already signed. This is not a legal contract.

Physicians are not required to have a discussion with their patients to obtain their consent and sometimes rely on written forms that the patient is handed and expected to read and sign on the spot. Unfortunately, the information on these forms can be difficult to understand—especially when one is anxious. Some health plans and physicians make use of DVD or computer-based programs to explain procedures and risks that can be completed prior to the procedure date. It is worth inquiring whether such a service is available to you.

Whether you have just read the consent form or you have talked with your doctor, if you do not feel that you fully understand what is going to happen to you when you get this procedure or that you are not sure that you know enough to weigh the risks and benefits, ask to discuss these questions with your physician before you go ahead.

One way to make sure that you fully understand what you are consenting to is to repeat back to your physician in your own words what you understand about each of the six points in the "informed" section. That way, if you have misunderstood something or forgotten to factor it in to your consent, your physician will be able to clarify or remind you about the full range of relevant information you should consider.

CHAPTER 7

What Will I Do about Work?

Your aim is to keep your job for the foreseeable future: it is a source of income and often the source of health insurance.

The best thing about all this is that I had a job to go to. I didn't miss anything and it was hard but I was so grateful that I had my work to do.
—Supreme Court Justice Sandra Day O'Connor, addressing the
National Coalition of Cancer Survivorship, 1994

WHAT ARE YOU GOING TO DO about your job? The right answer is that you don't know yet.

Maybe you feel like quitting tomorrow. Maybe you'll manage to take care of this whole crisis without missing a full day. Maybe you'll be in and out of work and then be on disability for a while and then quit. Maybe you don't really have a choice about this—you are going to be working until you can no longer drag yourself to your job.

You don't know now and you probably won't be able to tell for a while what this diagnosis means about how you are going to handle work in the long term. But as long as health care is so expensive and as long as most of us still receive our health insurance as a benefit through our workplaces, the safest short-term solution is to hang onto your job until you get a sense of how this condition will physically and mentally affect you.

This chapter is about a number of different aspects of work, but most important, it is about what you may want to think about and do today so that you don't close off any of your options about working in the future.

You probably won't be as productive as you usually are over the next few months, but even so, you may want to keep an eye out for what work offers you right now in addition to a paycheck and health insurance.

Your workplace probably offers some benefits—sick leave, unpaid leave, health insurance, and disability—and the state and federal government also provide important protections that should figure into your planning over the next few months. Being certain about what your benefits are will help relieve some worry and ensure you make use of what is available to you.

Because your condition will likely affect your job performance, it is worthwhile to think about how your diagnosis is going to affect your ability to do your job and your relationships with your co-workers and supervisors.

To Work or Not to Work?

For some people, the shock of bad health news or the condition (and its treatment) itself means that returning to work right now is simply not an option. For others, work quickly becomes background for the task of figuring out what to do next: you show up when you aren't gathering information and running between tests and appointments and treatments. And for some, work is like a lifeboat in a storm—the only place where events are familiar and predictable and you can maintain your sense of being a normal, functioning person like you were before.

When I asked people how they handled working during the period immediately following their diagnosis, they talked about four reasons to keep their jobs:

- I want to be distracted.

- I want people around me for support.

- My body has failed me but I am still able to contribute. I need the perspective work offers.

- I need the health insurance my job provides and my family needs my income.

Jane, fifty-three, an artist, felt that working was helpful:

> It focused me and helped me forget temporarily. What was I going to do, sit and look in the mirror? More likely, knowing me I would have just felt sorry for myself if I hadn't kept working.

"I got the news of my diagnosis and that I was going to have to have surgery immediately—that same day," said Dana, sixty-two, a foundation executive.

> I started frantically rearranging my work schedule in my head, not knowing what the surgery meant, what I was going to be able to do when. I had to mentally toss over my shoulder one thing after another. I finally decided that there was one part of my job that I love and that no one else can really do. It didn't involve travel, just talking on the phone. I decided I would do that and delegate everything else to others. This calmed me down immensely, for some reason.

"I didn't want anyone to put me in the sick role," said Don, fifty-two, an environmentalist.

> I was barely able to manage all the appointments and tests and not miss a full day of work. Sometimes I was just an automaton—I was numb. It upsets me that I was not able to be a help and a mentor like I usually am. Sometimes my young colleagues had to step in and help. It was not a generative time. But my company offers great health insurance and I have needed every bit of it.

But Hannah, thirty-seven, a teacher, ended up not being able to do her job and finally had to take a leave of absence during this period:

> I felt that all my energy was going into figuring out what to do about this when the doctors had no clue. It was a time of complete frustration.

My own experience with work after receiving three of my diagnoses was that it was the single most important thing that kept me from diving deep into the pit of despair. I think I thought that if I could still think, if I could still write, then somehow I still was okay.

I remember lying on the couch with that kind of fatigue that makes your very molecules cry out for rest, forcing myself to read, to take notes, to write. No one told me I had to do it. I am certain that any deadline would have been extended, had I asked. I just needed to do something that, like a string on a kite, connected me to a part of my life where things were predictable and where I wasn't this mess of physical dysfunction.

The nature of your condition, its treatment, your personal situation, and characteristics of your work and workplace will influence what you eventually do about working over the long term. However, there are different ways to approach working in the next few months. Whatever approach you choose in the coming few weeks, at a minimum you need to inform the human resources or benefits administrator—the person who has the responsibility of handling health insurance, leave, and other benefits at your workplace—that you have a medical condition that may interfere with work. You need not specify the diagnosis. That person may be able to help you shape an interim plan and help you think about your options.

How Can My Employer Be Helpful?

The fear that employers will respond punitively to a life-altering diagnosis is not borne out in the scientific literature, although anecdotes about worst-case scenarios abound. In fact, people generally do not experience discrimination or lose their jobs or their insurance following a serious diagnosis. Thomas Chirikos, a researcher at the Moffitt Cancer Center and Research Institute at the University of South Florida, who studies employment patterns in relation to cancer, speculates that the news coverage of incidents where people have been treated badly lead people to overestimate their risk of losing their job and insurance when ill.

I interviewed people with serious diagnoses and their loved ones about their experiences with work during this period. I talked with supervisors and employees of people who were sick and with human resources professionals from small, midsized, and large organizations. For the most part, I did not hear bad stories.

I heard about employers who bent the rules far beyond their own stated policies in order to help people in distress—both for those with the diagnosis and those caring for them. I heard about supervisors and employers who were generous and supportive, and about colleagues who assumed others' responsibilities and who helped out at work and at home.

But Lou Yaeger, executive director of Catastrophic Health

Planners, Inc., has heard a lot about the other response: "Some companies will take care of you beautifully and others will cut you off as soon as you cough. Be careful of what you disclose and know what you are required to disclose. Your employer has its own agenda and you aren't it."

You know your workplace. You know how your employer has treated other people with serious illnesses in themselves and their families.

You are not required to disclose the nature of your condition to anyone at work. Saying that you—or someone in your family—has a "serious medical condition" is enough to trigger the Family and Medical Leave Act and short-term disability provisions. If a letter from your doctor is required to invoke these protections, ask him to use this language as well.

Use your judgment and if you are at all concerned, err on the side of caution. Then you can change your mind and disclose more later if you want to.

WHAT ARE THE BASIC BENEFITS AND PROTECTIONS I SHOULD ASK ABOUT?

There are seven benefits that are relevant to you during these first few weeks after you have learned of a serious medical condition. You need to know about them because you may be in and out of work unpredictably for the foreseeable future. You want to have maximum flexibility without endangering your job. Plus, you should make use of those benefits you have earned and for which you have paid.

Paid leave: You need to know how much you have. What are the conditions for using it? Do you need to inform your supervisor in advance? Can you use it on an hourly basis?

Sick leave: Do you have this kind of leave? Does it accumulate? If so, how much do you have? What are the conditions for using it? Do you need a physician's note? Can you use it on an hourly basis? Can your co-workers donate their sick leave to you?

Unpaid leave: What are the terms for using unpaid leave? What kind of notification is required or can you just take it and have it classified as unpaid later?

Flextime: If your workplace allows flextime, you may be able to re-arrange your work to accommodate your medical appointments or later on, your treatment.

Health benefit: Knowing what your health plan or health insurance does and doesn't cover will relieve a little anxiety. See chapter 8 for an approach to learning only what you need to know right now about your health benefit.

Short-term disability: You may have elected to pay for this or your company may have done so. Employers vary in how, when, and who makes this decision to invoke your coverage under short-term disability insurance.

Family and Medical Leave Act (FMLA): If your workplace employs at least fifty employees and you have worked there for more than a year, you are probably eligible for the benefits provided by FMLA. As long as you are talking about the immediate term, it is a powerful tool based on a simple law: you have to demonstrate that you or a family member has a "serious medical condition"—then you are entitled to up to twelve weeks of unpaid leave without losing your job. Depending on how this leave is administered by your employers, it may offer you great flexibility in the coming months. FMLA covers leave for a person caring for an ill family member as well.

Even if you have a condition that you know now is going to disable you in the long-term, you can delay learning about long-term disability and the Americans with Disabilities Act until things calm down a little.

WHAT CAN YOU EXPECT FROM THE PERSON WHO ADMINISTERS THE BENEFITS?

The person responsible for human resources in your workplace will have a record of all the leave you have used and all that you are owed. She will be able to explain the employer's policies on sick leave and flextime. She will know about your health benefit—health plan or health insurance—and have some ideas about how to make the best use of it. And if you have access to Family and Medical Leave and short-term disability, this employee will describe how she can make use of these protections to maintain your job and your health insurance, especially during these first couple months until you have a better sense of what is going on.

Ann Pashby, a human resources manager at Rhode & Schwartz, Inc., in Maryland, said that her goal is to get employees as much of their normal pay for as long as they can.

Christina Donawa, a human resources administrator at the National Development and Research Institutes (NDRI), said, "Here is what people should expect from our human resources department: First, to advise you on informing your supervisor about your diagnosis. Second, to establish a plan to make sure you get all the benefits you are entitled to, to go over pay, accumulated vacation and sick leave and so on, so you know what is available. Third, to help you use those benefits—how to take advantage of the Family and Medical Leave Act provisions, short-term disability, Employee Assistance Program services, like family counseling and childcare. And fourth, if you are a member of a union, to remind you to explore what the union offers."

Don't be surprised, however, if your HR administrator sometimes seems to be learning the ropes along with you. You should expect that he has basic knowledge of your benefits and how they work, but you might be the first person to ever put some of these options into action, particularly if you work for a small business.

Dan Kohrman, an attorney and expert on age discrimination at AARP, first assumed that white-collar employers would be more responsive to serious medical conditions than blue-collar ones. However, Kohrman said, "My experience has shown me that white-collar employers are often at a loss about how to deal with people who are seriously ill because they have so many fewer of them—their employees are generally healthy. In blue-collar and unionized workplaces, on the other hand, people are more likely to be doing physical work and are more likely to get injured on the job, get back strain and so on. So their human resources departments are more likely to know how to handle disability, retirement considerations, light work accommodation, etc. It is not such a shock to the system for them to adjust to the challenge."

Here is some advice from human resources administrators working for employers including government agencies, a large state university, a Fortune 500 company, midsized blue- and white-collar firms, and a number of small workplaces:

> People are sometimes nervous or embarrassed to talk to their HR person but it works best if they do so right away. That way we can get started immediately addressing the employee's needs on a case-by-case basis and coordinate short-term disability and Family and Medical Leave Act protections so they work for each individual.
>
> Jude Sincoskie, human resources administrator,
> Rhode & Schwartz, Inc.

> When employees come in to HR for that first appointment after they've been diagnosed, I think it really helps if they bring their spouse or adult child or a friend. This is important information; it is complicated information and it is emotionally charged. Another pair of ears and someone to take notes really helps. I should mention, however, that at this point, no one should expect to remember all the ins and outs of short- and long-term disability and FMLA. There is time later to learn about this.
>
> Linda King, director of human resources,
> University of Oregon

> If an employee hasn't used her insurance much, she is probably not familiar with how to protect herself from getting caught in the fine-print rules, like precertification, the different costs of in-network and out-of-network doctors, and what affects the deductibles and copays. And she probably doesn't know about the other services the plan offers—the information on the Web site, the nurse advice line, the docfinder service, centers of excellence, and so on. I negotiated for those benefits and I know what is available. So when someone is going to start making use of them, I try to introduce employees to both the good parts and bad parts of the health plan.
>
> Loretta Graff, human resources associate,
> Carnegie Corporation of New York

> The flexibility of being at a place where people know you is invaluable. When you have just received a serious diagnosis, the last thing you

should think about is litigating to get the benefits you are entitled to. Even later on, if you feel that you have been treated unfairly, this is a bad idea. These are powerful tools that are better if used delicately, strategically, and minimally: get legal advice behind the scenes. Your general approach toward your employer should be not to antagonize but, rather, to meet them halfway, to propose choices, and to be reasonable.

Dan Kohrman, AARP attorney

This is not the time to change jobs. Hang on tight to the one you have! If through an accident of bad timing, you are about to leave a job with health benefits, talk with the human resources person to plan out how to manage this. COBRA is a federal act that gives you the option of paying [employer's negotiated price] for your existing coverage for up to eighteen months after leaving [if you participate in a group plan and your company has more than twenty employees]. Seriously: if this is your situation, do it. It will be hard to find other coverage at this point in your illness.

Christina Donawa, human resources administrator,

NDRI

One final piece of advice: You know that notebook you are using to take notes in about your doctor visits? Use the same notebook to take notes on every conversation you have with the human resources or benefits administrator. It's easy to forget things and you may need to refer to the dates and substance of your conversation later on.

Advice about Maximizing the Benefits
of Your Benefits

The person who administers the benefits in your workplace is someone you should be able to trust with personal information about yourself. In most workplaces, this person is charged with maintaining the confidentiality of all employees, since she or he often has access to personnel records, including salary history, use of benefits, disciplinary action, and so on.

One of the things I tell newly diagnosed employees is that if you want your confidentiality protected, you need to say, "I am not ready to have this information shared." They shouldn't have to do this, since their confidentiality is protected by the privacy act (HIPAA). It is just a safe-guard and reminder to everyone about what they want.

Linda King, director of human resources, University of Oregon

If you have any questions about how the person who is in charge of benefits will treat your personal health information, you may want to clarify this prior to any further discussion of your situation. The benefits administrators I talked with were very certain about their responsibilities to maintain employee privacy, as part of their job description and their professional code. However, at smaller and less formal workplaces where the person administering the benefits may also answer the phone or have other responsibilities, it may be wise to check with this administrator about how he views his role.

"I work closely with supervisors to help manage their expectations of the worker, to try to help them get the resources they need so they don't take a blow, too—and so they don't pressure a sick worker to come back before he is ready," said Christina Donawa, of NDRI. "But I do this without disclosing the diagnosis unless the worker explicitly tells me that I can. In an ideal world, employees would come see me as soon as they learn they have a serious condition so we could talk about the pros and cons of letting their supervisor and co-workers know about it and, if so, how to tell them."

Linda King, of the University of Oregon, said that many people just go in to work and tell everybody their terrible news. "They are comfortable with their colleagues and know they will get lots of positive support. They forget that their diagnosis may upset some of their co-workers, may derail a promising career, or may be disruptive to others who will have to pick up the slack when they are absent. Their boss may not be pleased to be the last one to hear about the diagnosis, for example, or to have to adjust work assignments to make up for planned and unplanned absence. I understand why people don't think ahead at this point, by the way. It's our job to help them do so, though."

Remember: You are not required to disclose the nature of your condition to anyone at work.

How Will My Co-workers Be Affected by My Condition?

I actually didn't think much about this one way or the other until my most recent experience. I had gotten my preliminary diagnosis and two days later headed off to work. I found myself blurting out the news to a couple of my employees. But since I didn't really know what was going to happen and I was deep into envisioning worst–case scenarios, I kind of fell apart. My eyes welled up with tears and I couldn't speak. This frightened them. I think they thought I would quit soon, if not die, and that they would lose their jobs.

Was this really necessary? I don't know, and I don't know if this incident itself changed anything irretrievably, but it started me thinking about how telling people about what is going on with you sets off a cascade of reactions and consequences that bear thinking about.

Regardless of how you feel about your work and the people who do it with you, people are going to notice if you are not there, are not feeling well, or not producing as usual. It will affect your relationships with them whether or not you tell them the reason.

Many people I interviewed told their co–workers about their diagnoses and were surprised and touched by the support they received. They described being reassigned to do low priority routine work for a while to lessen their performance pressure; having colleagues volunteer to accompany them to every doctor visit; co–workers who drove three children to school and back; a leave donation effort that gave a single mom an extra three months at home to get back on her feet.

The stories are heartwarming. And people are often genuinely glad to be able to help.

A few things to consider, though:

You can *hope* for these kinds of responses but should not *expect* them. I also heard stories of co–workers who promised to help but didn't deliver; of workplaces where the condition was perceived as a personal weakness and resulted in marginalizing the employee; and about colleagues who were resentful when they were asked to pick up the work left undone due to illness.

Annette, fifty-nine, a human resources administrator herself, said that when she was diagnosed with HIV/AIDS, she found that handling her new diagnosis at work was hard:

> I met with each of the department heads and told them about the probable course of the disease. The people I worked with didn't have any experience with this disease, and it was new and frightening to them. Some people thought they could catch it from me. We ended up doing an educational piece on it for everyone. This experience has made me sympathetic. We try to work things out—legally or illegally, if we need to—to make it possible for people to get through tough times like this.

Nell, thirty-three, a lawyer, talked to her firm's HR person the same day she received her diagnosis:

> Then I told my supervisor and the people who were working for me that I just got some bad medical news and I had to get my balance and that I didn't know how this would affect my work. I didn't feel comfortable breaking down in front of them. It's a very cut-throat, high-pressure kind of place. I guess the news filtered out via others, but I only ever told a couple people what was going on—my supervisor and two colleagues.

"In my business, it doesn't matter how you feel," said Edward, forty-five, a cab driver.

> If you show up and do the work, you get paid. I just couldn't manage it some days but I kept going in until they let me go. I'd never been fired before but I needed the money and then the unemployment [insurance payments].

"Are you nuts?" said Noah, an investment banker.

> They still don't know at work. I wouldn't be able to bring in business. People wouldn't trust my abilities. They'd think less of me. I'd no longer be a promising young star. I will quit before I tell anyone there.

Barrie, forty-nine, a cancer researcher, sent an e-mail to everyone in her work group.

> I thought it would be simpler. I said, "This is my diagnosis and this is how I'm feeling and I hope you will support me through this." And they did.

Your illness is central to you, but the wheels of your workplace grind on. In other words, your boss is still responsible for making sure all the work gets done. A senior government official who has a lot of experience with employees who have catastrophic conditions explained, "As a supervisor, your first thought is what you can do to help, what the organization can do to help. Then you have to figure out how to make do. People pitch in and are not grudging about this. Usually a few close colleagues organize this, though you have to be careful about people feeling coerced to join. After about a week, the supervisor starts to worry about logistics in the short- and mid-term. It's hard to find a back burner for a front-line person. You want to preserve the sick employee's place in the work group, but you have to meet your numbers."

The studies that have been done on this topic suggest that it is unlikely that you will be fired because of your illness. But holding on to your job and maintaining a good relationship with your supervisor requires some effort. "When an employee is in and out because of an illness, you want him to come in and tell you how much he can do. It is difficult for the supervisor to plan how to work around. Knowing when the person is going to feel okay is the critical issue for the supervisor and for the team," said a real estate manager.

Well, when *are* you going to feel okay? You would probably like to know the answer to this question, too. "If there is a human resources department, it may be able to help by finding temporary help or negotiating the politics of hiring," said Linda King, of the University of Oregon. "But there is no substitute for maintaining open communication between employee and supervisor. Employees often want to believe they can produce like they did when they were well. They don't realize that it can be more problematic for the supervisor when they promise to be there and then don't show up than it would be if they just said not to count on them for the next week."

CHAPTER 8

Pay for Care

Your aim is to make the best possible use of all available assets, get the care you need and protect yourself and your family financially.

I did not expect that the financial side of this diagnosis would be so complicated—at least not to this degree or that it would happen with every procedure. It was so upsetting and it took so much energy. I would characterize it as almost as upsetting as the disease—it was like adding insult to injury.

Clyde, 39—administrator

I HAD JUST TURNED TWENTY and was still lying in the intensive care unit a week after surgery, fully wired for light and sound, being shipped once a day to the basement of the hospital to get a massive dose of radiation to my chest. I was mostly sleeping—and distraught when I wasn't. Through the fog of drugs and the moans of the burn patient in the next cubicle, I had overheard a conversation between my parents—something about, "I don't think our insurance covers this."

And there I was, with each breath of oxygen spending my brothers' college funds, each radiation treatment diminishing my family's life savings, each bag of saline using up the grocery money.

I wondered if they would be better off if I didn't make it through this crisis. What should I do? What *could* I do? How could I ever make up to them for impoverishing them? I was twenty years old and so, so sick! And I felt that I held the economic future of my family in my weak hands.

I have since then assumed that part of the reason a serious diagnosis is devastating is that it forces you to weigh the consequences of your life and death in deeply practical terms as well as in existential ones. So it was a little surprising that when

I interviewed health professionals for this book, many of them discouraged my intention to write about finances and work and insurance. Their impression was that people are so overwhelmed when they get a serious diagnosis that they really don't think about those things and that they are willing to do whatever it takes to get the care they need. But these financial concerns cut across age, class, and cultural lines.

Maybe it's just that people don't talk to health professionals about this part of their lives because the disease and treatment take up so much room in their common conversations. But I can tell you from my own experience and that of those I interviewed for this book these concerns are real, they are central and they are agonizing. The prospect of losing one—or the only—source of income or the threat of spending precious savings that guarantee your future as well as your family's add to one's sense of panic, distress, and guilt during this uncertain time.

Drita Taraila, a social worker at the Abramson Cancer Center at the University of Pennsylvania noted, "The saying is true: the whole family gets the diagnosis. Only one person gets the surgery and the drugs, but the trauma visited on the family is palpable."

This chapter addresses two aspects of trying to limit the financial impact of serious illness: making good use of insurance and the need to take a look at your financial status in preparation for whatever is to come. It may be hard to concentrate on these topics right now and it is probably premature to make any quick changes, but there are a few key things that you will want to consider.

The first section of this chapter offers a framework for thinking about your health insurance as you move through the coming weeks: it will allow you to read the description of your health plan or insurance and pick out only the parts of the policies you need to know about *right now*. It also presents some basic rules of thumb that may be useful as you start racking up the bills for consultations and tests.

The second section discusses a few basic practical actions for financial planning that you can take now to anticipate the challenge ahead, regardless of your financial resources or whether you are covered by health insurance.

Three Things You Need to Know about Your Health Insurance Right Now

Pretend that you have no health insurance and are not a member of a health plan. Instead, you have a rich uncle who loves you very much and who has an infinite amount of money. If you get really sick, you just go to whatever doctor you choose and that uncle will pay for all those consultations and treatments and drugs and hospitalizations you need.

Every month you have been paying for health-care insurance because, in all likelihood, you don't have a rich uncle and you knew that if you had a catastrophic illness you would need financial help. Unfortunately, health insurance doesn't operate like a rich uncle, regardless of whether it is provided by the government (Medicare or Medicaid), your employer, or your union, or is purchased by you as an individual.

Rather, it works by placing limits on three different areas of health care delivery, says Ray Werntz, a longtime human resources executive in the private sector. A health benefit lays out three categories of rules of engagement between individuals who need health services and the professionals and institutions that provide them. While plans vary widely, you can generally expect that your plan will define:

- *Which providers can deliver health-care services*

- *The ground rules for interacting with them,* for example, do you need to be referred to a specialist?

- *What is covered,* or what services and tests and drugs will be paid for and which will be excluded?

The main thing you need to know now are the specific rules of *your* health benefit in each of these areas, whether you participate in Medicare or Medicaid or are a member of an HMO or other type of health plan. Only then can you make a conscious choice about when to make use of the resources of your benefit plan and when to take the financial hit of going outside it by choosing doctors or hospitals not preferred by your plan, by ignoring the procedural rules, or by seeking treatments excluded from coverage.

Which providers? Your health plan may have a list of doctors, hospitals, and health-care facilities with whom it contracts and pays discounted rates. Or it may specify, as does Medicare, that it will pay almost all providers, but only a set amount.

> I have a preferred provider plan and I used doctors on the list, even though I saw a couple of them who weren't when I was being worked up. When you finally find—or get referred to—the person who is going to treat you, it may be someone you are going to go to for the rest of your life, and you need to be able to afford it.
>
> Suzanne, 36—economist

Right now you need to know:

- Which doctors, hospitals, and health-care facilities participate in your plan that specialize in diagnosing and treating your disease

- What your copay is (how much you pay for every visit or service) and your deductible (what you pay before the plan pays the rest), and the differences in cost for those providers who are in your plan's network versus those who are not

- How much it will cost you if the specialist you choose is not approved by your health plan or does not take your insurance

Human resources manager Ann Pashby pointed out that most plans have an out-of-pocket maximum. "You can only be asked to pay up to a certain amount of your own money in copayments. Even though it seems like a hunk of money to go through—like $2,000—crossing that threshold can provide welcome relief."

What are the ground rules for interacting? Your health plan has set in place procedures to make sure that you get the right care for your condition or get the right tests that are affordable to you and the plan. Often, these controls feel to us as though the health plan is trying to withhold needed services or care. Always, they feel like an extra hassle.

Right now, you need to know:

- If you are required to be referred by your primary care provider to a specialist

- What is required of you when you need to go to the emergency room? For example, do you need to call your plan within twenty-four hours to let them know that you have been there?

- If diagnostic and staging procedures, such as MRIs or CAT scans, must be approved by your plan. This is often called "precertification" or "preauthorization," and whether this is your responsibility to do or if the staff of the physician who ordered the test will do it, paying close attention to this can minimize delays and avoid unforeseen expenses.

- If a procedure must be done at an outpatient facility or hospital that participates in your plan.

What is covered? During the diagnostic and early treatment stages of most conditions, most procedures and tests are covered by a health plan if you choose to receive the standard medical treatment for your condition. Coverage becomes more of a concern with later stages of treatment—particularly if standard treatments are not working and more experimental methods seem promising.

The key determinant of what is covered is whether or not a service is *medically necessary*, as determined by the plan, usually based on a careful reading of the medical literature by researchers and professionals. It may be important at some later point to look into who decides medical necessity for your plan and whether you can appeal denial of coverage on this basis.

Right now, however, you need to know:

- If your plan includes a pharmacy benefit and if so, how to use it and how much it will cost. Even though you have pharmacy coverage, you may pay significantly more for drugs if you buy them at your local pharmacy than through a specific mail-order pharmacy, for example. You may still choose to go to your local drugstore during this time because over the next few weeks, you are more likely to need a prescription filled this afternoon. But your plan's mail-order pharmacy may have a fast turnaround service, and, if you are familiar with how it works, it may be more convenient and cheaper to use it.

- Whether your plan distinguishes generic from name-brand drugs in its reimbursement procedures to encourage the use of lower-cost generic drugs when they are appropriate for your condition.

You may decide that you are not going to be bound by the limits that your health plan imposes. You may decide to consult physicians who do not take any insurance at all or work with a health-care provider such as an alternative healer, for example. The point is *not* that you *must* stay within the limits but rather that you should *choose* when you want to exceed them, recognizing that there are financial consequences to doing so.

So here's a suggestion. Get out a description of your health benefit. Read it with the sole aim of finding out your plan's rules and practices regarding these three topics. It should take you no more than half an hour. Do this again in a couple days to see if you come up with the same answers.

The reason to do it again is that you are learning so much so fast about how to get health care right now—and you may not even realize that you are—that the information will look different the second time through.

If you have questions about what you have read, call the plan. The number is right there on the cover of the booklet. Or ask others for help understanding the ground rules.

Rules of Thumb for Using Your Health Plan

It is wise to start with the assumption that your relationship with your health plan or insurer will be cooperative and informative—that getting the care you need is a concern you have in common and that you are going to collaborate on solving this problem. You should keep good records about your health care—and about your calls to your health plan—regardless of whether this assumption proves true.

Actually, I remind myself of this assumption before any phone call to my health plan or to hospital and clinic billing departments. Chances are that I won't talk to the same person I talked to the last time when I might have ummm…lost it, shall we say, and I have the opportunity to start over, to try to forge an alliance with this new person who has answered the phone and who will join with me so that together we can solve the problem I am calling about.

Here is a little guidance about things you should do as you are getting accustomed to frequent contact with health-care deliverers:

- ALWAYS carry your current insurance card(s) with you. (See chapter 6 for suggestions about what information you should take with you to all appointments.)

- The printing on most cards is absurdly small. Make—or ask someone else to make—a readable copy of both sides that includes your identification numbers, the telephone numbers, and the address of the company.

- Read the back of your insurance card. Note particularly the telephone numbers for precertification, emergency treatment, and questions about coverage.

- Whether or not they are on the list, always ask a physician if he or she accepts your insurance when you call to make an appointment. If the doctor does not, find out how much the consultation will cost.

- Do not assume that when a physician who participates in your health plan or accepts your insurance refers you to another physician that this new doctor will also take your insurance.

- Always check with the doctor who orders a test to see if it requires precertification from your health plan. If it does, make sure that this has been done, whether you do it yourself or your doctor's office does it.

- Know which doctors are available to you within the network (at a lower out-of-pocket cost). Take your provider book with you to appointments if you expect to be referred to another specialist. Ask your doctor to make a referral from the list. If you are covered by Medicare or Medicaid, ask the doctor's staff if patients covered by your program are accepted at that office, *before* you set up an appointment. It is very rare these days that there is only one place or one person who can do the procedure and provide the care.

- Every single time you see a doctor, there is a charge, whether you have to pull out your credit card at the end of the appointment or the doctor bills your insurer directly. In addition, you—or your insurance—will pay for every lab report, x-ray, and pill. This generates a lot of paper and you are going to see much of it. Often the insurance claims arrive at the same time as the bills. It can be confusing when you receive both simultaneously and are unable to match the claim with the bill and the event. Keep all bills and claims statements. Try to match dates and services. If you have questions, then call the customer service number of your insurance carrier. Keep a careful record of date, time, notes, and who you talked with for every conversation.

- If you need surgery and your surgeon accepts your insurance, always make sure that you know what is billed through the hospital—and whether the hospital takes your insurance. Ask whether the other physicians involved (the assisting surgeon, anesthesiologist) accept your insurance.

- Here are a few practical things you need to know about interacting with the customer service side of your health plan:

  — Customer service representatives do not have access to your medical record.

  — You can contact most health plans by mail or by telephone and often by e-mail as well.

  — Any contacts you have with customer service at your health plan will be documented so you shouldn't have to start at the very beginning of your story every time you call. You should also document each interaction as well.

  — Customer service representatives can only answer questions about your benefits and are the wrong people to ask about medical concerns.

Taking Care of Business

Whether or not you have health insurance, this diagnosis is likely to pose a threat—the size of which is as yet unknown—to your financial stability.

How you will absorb whatever hits are coming depends on your current financial position and your ability to act cautiously and thoughtfully. Because things may be happening very quickly now and you may not know yet what treatment you need or what the impact of the disease and the treatment will be on your ability to work, much less how complete your insurance coverage will be, you may find yourself reluctant to think very far ahead. And in the absence of a sense of where your financial assets and liabilities are, it is easy to let your imagination take you through financial worst-case scenarios that tear you apart.

All things being equal, then, it is worthwhile to take some time to look over your current situation so that you know what you have to work with.

"Most people don't have a handle on their complete financial picture on a day-to-day basis," said Mario Pitchon, of Strategies for Wealth Management and Creation. "Take an inventory of what you have and what you owe so you can protect your assets and know what you have that you can draw upon. Don't make any sudden moves. Consider consulting with a financial professional and family members who can help you sort out where you stand."

> You know how everyone always says to take a buddy to the doctor with you? Well, I think you need a buddy to help you get your bills organized. Especially at the beginning when whole rafts of them come in and you are so upset anyway.
>
> Clyde, 36—administrator

"You may have to plan for an hour from now, rather than a week from now," said Lou Yager, of Catastrophic Health Planners, Inc. "This is what these devastating diagnoses are like: first you think about what you want to accomplish in the next twenty minutes. It is a long, organizational process that just won't quit. And for each person it is different."

He continued, "Start here: what is your immediate goal? To stay alive. Then what? If there is anything that pops into your head as a problem that is not resolved, now is the time to put it on the list. Once you address it, you can put it aside—you unload the plate and it will help you calm down. Are you worried about finances? Health care for the kids? Your treatment expenses? Paying for your funeral? Set up your list."

At the early stage of a diagnosis when so much is as yet unknown, your aim might be to do just these two things: First, get a clear picture of your current assets and liabilities, and second, put together a list of the things that you will need to address, given your worst-case scenario. Then you may want to consider going over both with a financial professional or a disinterested family member to begin to detail your options.

Here is additional advice from financial experts about how, even at this early stage, you might prepare for the uncertain financial demands ahead:

- If you suspect or know that there are going to be times when you are not going to be functioning fully in the next few months, make a list of payments that you know will need to be made: your usual bills as well as some that are less regular, like life, auto, liability, and property insurance. If you will be receiving treatment away from your home, make arrangements with the post office to forward your mail. A good broker will notify you of an impending insurance lapse but you can't depend on this.

- Everything is negotiable: hospital bills, doctor bills, your credit card bills. Few people and companies want to go to court and most will be willing to talk with you to find ways to avoid doing so. But you may not be the right person to negotiate for yourself, especially if you are feeling weak or confused from the disease or treatment. This kind of negotiation takes some skill. If you feel that you can't engage in this type of decision-making because you are too sick or you don't know how, you need to find the right person. Ask for help from a savvy friend or family member or a financial professional.

- "If you don't have insurance and can't afford the cost of a visit, you can talk to the doctor about a possible discount," said Barrie, forty–nine, a cancer researcher. "Remember though, when you ask for a discount, you are *not* saying 'I'm only worthy of second–rate care.' Rather, you are saying 'I can't afford your fees. I am as interested in getting good care as the next guy. Can we talk about what we can do to make it affordable for me?' Then let the doctor suggest a solution. Hopefully he will suggest paying less or paying over time."

- Some doctors and hospitals are willing to set up interest–free installment payment plans. Inquire whether this might be an option.

- Many loans for cars, houses, and credit cards that were given out years ago had disability insurance on them that was given as a benefit of the card. Check to see if you have disability insurance on your liabilities. If you have it and you become disabled and are unable to work, you will not be responsible for the debt. Often people are not aware of this. Check your loans and credit card policies to see whether you have this kind of coverage.

- There are a growing number of nonprofit organizations that provide assistance to individuals and families facing a devastating illness in the form of help sorting through their financial options, applying for Medicaid or Social Security, negotiating medical fees, and planning to absorb the financial impact of a serious illness. See appendices F, G, and H for more information on these organizations.

LEGAL DOCUMENTS YOU NEED RIGHT NOW

Every financial professional I interviewed mentioned the importance of having up–to–date legal documents in case you are unable to make decisions for yourself, such as a will, medical power of attorney, health–care proxy, and an advance directive.

"Hey! I'm not dying yet!" you say. Well, then this is, indeed, the right time for you to complete these tasks.

- You are acutely aware of the fragility of your life right now.

- You just looked over your current assets and liabilities and know where you stand financially.

- While you may not know what kind of care you *do* want if you become very ill, you probably know what you *don't* want, and you risk the latter if you don't assert yourself through these legal tools.

- You know that if you don't make some clear decisions now, your loved ones will be greatly limited in carrying out your wishes and your outdated will is going to enrich your ex-wife or allow the state to distribute your assets.

Dean, a professor, said that he had been "lazy" about doing an advance directive and medical power of attorney. "They make you do it at the hospital before you have surgery and I hated doing it so fast and thoughtlessly. I wished I had done it sooner than moments before I was wheeled into surgery."

See appendix H for a description of the basic documents you should have completed, resources that provide guidance about doing so, the requirements of your state for each one, and information about how to ensure that your wishes are acted upon.

Taking care of this business is hard. You are forced to imagine your death and its impact on your friends and family. But as painful as it is to think about this and to take these actions, these legal protections are acts of generosity. They lift the burden of difficult decisions from those you love.

Act now.

CHAPTER 9

Find a Little Relief

Your aim is to find get some relief from the constant stress of this new diagnosis so you can gather the strength you need to participate in your treatment and in your life.

Nothing anyone says or does can change this diagnosis and what it means for me. I am *uncomfortable*. Literally. There is not a moment when I am not dreading what is to come.

Chris, 38—archeologist

THE INTENSITY OF YOUR DISTRESS may wax and wane as you recover from the surprise of your diagnosis and start nailing down the details of what you must do next. But for many of us, the weight of our situation is inescapable and we long for some moments of relief.

I asked the people I interviewed about what helped them to calm down, what gave them a break from their anxiety so that they could regroup a bit and find some perspective about the future. They were deeply sympathetic with the readers of this book. They know how difficult this time is, and they each expressed a desire that others might benefit from their experience. They talked about a range of approaches that were more or less helpful during the time when there were in deepest distress. These are described here, organized into several general strategies for finding relief during the first days after a devastating diagnosis.

You already know what works best to help you calm down. You have a lifetime of experience in this. But in case your familiar ways of regaining your composure are not working, consider these.

Maintain a Routine

One way people talked about stemming the feeling that their world was spinning out of control during the first few weeks after a devastating diagnosis was to hold on to as much of their daily routines as they could.

It requires some effort to get up at the same time you always have and eat your usual breakfast while watching the *Today* show, even though you aren't going to work, aren't hungry, and have more pressing concerns than the state of the world or the latest celebrity cookbook. But it may help you feel less disoriented. Marking the passage of time with regular meals and routine activities that do not physically or emotionally tax you can provide some small relief from the uncertainty you are experiencing.

> I organized my life so that I was as active and normal as possible. I got up, took a shower, kept the house neat. I couldn't read, but I could sit and walk. I couldn't sleep and couldn't nap, so I was exhausted. But I did little tasks like clean up my desk when I felt like it.
>
> Allan, 75—retired physician

Keeping up with routines may also be important for your family—particularly if you have children living with you. Regardless of how much children know about what is going on, they need to feel that home is safe and predictable. Even if you know that their future security is threatened by your illness, you will be able to comfort them now by maintaining the rhythms and rituals of home.

This does not mean denying that you are facing a crisis or ignoring the need to respond to it. It means doing the best you can to make sure that the rest of the family doesn't join you in feeling wildly out of control. Do this by keeping food in the house, maintaining usual bedtimes, getting everyone to school on time, and having familiar supervision. And it means taking care of yourself by asking others to take on some of these tasks if you feel like it and can arrange it.

Depending on how fragile you feel right now, you may decide that, once you have fulfilled the demands of appointments and information collection, you can only preserve one part of your routine: breakfast with the newspaper, for example. Or a cup of tea and a cookie in the afternoon. "You need to conserve your energy right now," said psychiatric clinical nurse specialist Janet Baradell, "Ask yourself if this is a one-event day or a two-event day."

Seek Distraction

Norman Cousins wrote a book recounting his experience with severe spinal arthritis in 1979, and in it described watching funny movies for hours on end, finding that that laughter really helped him feel better. People I talked to noted the same thing. If they could find the right thing to distract them, doing so allowed them to take a brief vacation from their despair.

> I had about six weeks of uncertainty between my tentative diagnosis and the confirmation of a different, much scarier diagnosis. I sent out an e-mail to all my friends and said, "Please send me anything that is funny—books, movies, cards." I got tons. I would watch as many as two movies each night. And I was like a child waiting for the mail—it gave me something to look forward to.
>
> Clyde, 39—administrator

> I spent a lot of time playing with my three-year-old granddaughter. Children are right there with you at that age and they demand your attention—plus they know when your mind wanders. We read the same books over and over, played at making lunch hundreds of times. It was good for me to stop thinking about myself and great to have that precious time with her.
>
> Adele, 70—retired teacher

Cindy, thirty-six, a homemaker, said that one of the best things she did a few weeks after being diagnosed was to attend a local comedy night.

> We had already purchased tickets for it, so we went. The comedians were great and it felt good to laugh instead of cry for an evening. I would recommend seeing a funny movie, reading a light book, anything to distract you from your fear and sadness.

Me? I tried reading but couldn't focus and television drove me mad. Listening to music made me weep. Finally I realized that playing the piano gave me hours when I didn't think about myself or my condition at all. I'm not a good enough pianist to daydream while I play. I have to concentrate, so playing meant I could have whole blocks of time that I wasn't thinking about what might happen next.

Spend Time with Friends

There is something about friends—as distinct from family—that make them unique valuable assets in finding relief. Somehow, because friends are just a little more removed from you, they can empathize with you, can sympathize with your situation, but they are not there in that deep pit with you. Unlike your closest family members, they are not spending all their time concentrating on learning about the disease and scheduling doctors. Nope. They are still coaching little league, going to work, fixing the car. And that can make all the difference.

Friends are people who knew you before you had this diagnosis. Their mere presence can remind you of the rich life you had and shared with them before you became preoccupied with this disease. They can take some of the pressure off by helping out with day-to-day tasks such as mowing your lawn or driving you home after a test.

> I've had great support from my friends. Someone arranged for me to get a flu shot. One friend still calls every day just to check in. They got together and organized it so that someone brought dinner over every night for a month.
>
> Sarah, 60—homemaker

But friends are also willing to treat you like the person you were before you got the diagnosis.

I decided very early on to get a wig in anticipation of losing my hair. A friend came along and we goofed around, just like we were trying on clothes at Bloomingdales. And then we went out for ice cream. We didn't talk about what was going on, particularly. We just had a nice, normal Saturday afternoon. It just made it less awful.

Nell, 33—lawyer

I have played poker every Tuesday with the same guys for decades. Just the fact that I could go there and someone would say, "How's it going?" and I had the chance to say "Fine" or "Terrible" made all the difference. They all knew what I was going through but I didn't have to talk about it. No one treated me like I was sick or damaged—no preferential treatment. The cards fell wherever they fell. I won some and I lost some.

Andrew, 63—manager

The difference between conversations you have with friends and those you might have with people who also have your disease is that you have a whole web of experiences and interests and history in common with your friends.

Over time you may build friendships with others that are based on the common experience of having your disease, and it may be that because coping with your condition takes up so much of your available energy—and because your friends really don't understand its effect on you—you will gravitate to those with whom you share this unique knowledge and leave your friends behind for a while.

Relax Physically

What do you usually do when you want to physically relax? Have you been doing those things since you got your diagnosis?

Many people report having physical symptoms—headache, back pain, twitchy eyes, upset stomach—in the days following their diagnosis. These are common when people are under stress but they can easily be mistaken for symptoms of your condition, and that can be disconcerting.

One way to counter the effects of physical stress during this time is to use the approaches that you know have worked in the past to reduce it. Some people know they need to find some physical relief from the pressure of their bad news and try new things, like drinking themselves into oblivion or getting a massage. Obviously, the latter is preferable to the former.

> Overall, I'm a healthy person, but I'm a teacher and am around a lot of kids and germs. I took a half-time medical leave from my job and used that time to confirm my diagnosis, find a really good doctor, and go to the gym to relieve the stress. I also started taking swing dancing lessons.
>
> Hannah, 37

> After the first week, my doctor gave me a prescription for sleeping pills. You need to be able to sleep and you need to be clear-headed and hear what people are saying to you.
>
> Fania, 68—retired receptionist

Mark, forty-four, a writer, recounted how his father, a retired marine, rejected the doctor's advice to begin taking medication that might slow the progression of the disease:

> Instead he began intense physical training which he hoped would provide the strength necessary to fight the disease. He approached it with the same determination he approached everything in his life.

Read and Write

Reading was absolutely essential in finding relief for some people and completely useless for others. And this preference didn't seem to fall along predictable lines. People who considered themselves very book-oriented couldn't take in the meaning of the printed word, whereas some people who usually preferred television or the Internet found that their ability to control the pace of information they were absorbing made reading more attractive.

Of course, there were those who found relief in mastering the current knowledge about their condition:

I own every book that was printed on MS and there are about four sentences in each that were useful.

Terry, 35—foundation executive

We simply devoured everything that might possibly be relevant, from WebMD and other science sites to find out about my disease, to books on spiritual and emotional healing. We felt like we were on top of the situation. If there was something we could know that would make a difference, we were going to find it.

Eleanor, 64—consultant

I really wanted to know how other people handled this. I tried to find a support group by reading other people's accounts of their experience.

Marilyn, 59—minister

If you think reading might help, take yourself to one of the big bookstores or your library and spend a couple of hours browsing.

You'll find things that you definitely don't want anywhere near you, but by the same token, you may find yourself really attracted by some other, unlikely ones. Don't just look in the self-help section and don't just look at books about your disease. Look at all the health books and then look at the spirituality shelves if it attracts you, and in the religion section. I would spend afternoons at the bookstore poking around. I found some real treasures that lifted my spirits immeasurably.

Clyde, 39—administrator

I found reading helpful, but only in waiting rooms. My choice was fiction books whose most notable characteristic was that they were long. I wanted plots that were slow-moving and complicated so I couldn't speed my way through and be left sitting there with another hour to wait with only old *People* magazines to look at.

Many people I talked to tried but failed to find relief in reading.

David, sixty-four, an environmentalist, received seven copies of *It's Not about the Bike* by Lance Armstrong:

I'm sure my friends thought it would be inspirational for me to read about him—you know, it would give me hope and courage—and also help me figure out how to cope. But I'll tell you, I read the first couple chapters and quit. It sounded so awful and it scared me. What was I going to do—not go through with the treatment? I have my own map of suffering and it scares me enough to think about that.

It was very difficult for me to read and focus, but I could listen to books on tape—Harry Potter, meditation tapes, tapes on the mind/body connection, visualization tapes. I found that there was a fine line between blaming myself for my disease versus being able to turn around my fear. Listening helped me.

Barrie, 49—cancer researcher

My son bought me the definitive book about my disease—what it was and how I could take control of it. It was huge. After I finally got a confirmed diagnosis, I came home and tried to read it. I would start reading and start crying. After a couple of days, my husband finally said, "Don't read the book—it's okay."

Sarah, 60—homemaker

Actually, among the people I interviewed, more of them turned away from reading during this period than found refuge in it. Among those who did not read, a number of people mentioned feeling that the only things they thought they should or could read were books related to their condition, and that these books scared them. They often talked about feeling this way about books in which famous (and not-so-famous) people describe their experiences with the diagnosis and treatment of their diseases and the insights they discovered. The same was true for self-help books about the long-term management of a condition. Many people were simply unready to absorb this kind of information yet. They said that such books were more interesting later on, after the shock had worn off—when they had accepted that they had this disease and were starting to adjust their lives to it.

The books mentioned by those who found reading helpful fell into four categories (apart from the "mysteries," "trashy novels," and "historical fiction" genres):

- Religious texts, particularly the Bible

- Books about finding meaning in the midst of crisis

- Books that discuss how crises are viewed within a faith or religious tradition

- Books about strengthening your body (diet and nutrition, exercise, complementary treatments)

I heard similar hot or cold responses to the idea of writing at this time:

> I kept a daily diary of what was going on and my emotions—what I did, how I felt, who came by, what they brought. Then I would read it back and I could see progress.
>
> Jerry, 59—retired nurse

> I chronicled everything so I wouldn't forget. I had heard from others that I would forget this—that it was too painful. Why not take pictures? Why not write? You think you will never forget this, but you do. So I have pictures of me bald with all these needles in me—sometimes I look at it to see my reconstruction. I use it as a reference.
>
> Barrie, 49—researcher

> People gave us beautiful journals. There is not a word in any of them. I was too sick and my partner was so exhausted from dealing with this that she couldn't write.
>
> Carmen, 37—nurse

Explore or Affirm Spirituality

For many people, a devastating diagnosis brings them hard up against the meaning of their life and the possibility—even inevitability—of their death. Faith in God can be of great comfort or can seem like a betrayal at this time. For many of the people I interviewed, their religion was their main source of strength and sustenance while they were responding to the crisis. It was not a choice they made to "help them cope" but rather their faith is a force inextricable from their daily lives.

Others, however, had less intense involvement with this aspect of life. Some had historical conflicts with religion, and some had no use for it altogether. By raising the idea of exploring or affirming one's spirituality, I am not suggesting that people turn to God in an instrumental way but, rather, I recognize the impulse of many people to turn to a higher power when faced with a life-threatening event. Among those who talked with me, a good number who did not consider themselves particularly spiritual and who were not affiliated with a religion prayed or sought out a minister, priest, or rabbi during the days just following their diagnosis, and others sought the fellowship of a faith community. Most reported that it helped them feel more grounded and calmer.

> I called my rabbi in distress two days before I had surgery. She gave me a book of psalms for people who are in trouble. She came to visit me in the hospital and she asked me to read a couple of the psalms. Up to then I hadn't been able to cry or let go.
>
> Sarah, 60—homemaker

> We belong to a close-knit congregation and I cannot describe how important the love and support and attention was to us. We felt we were walking through fire and they were right there with us every step of the way. It was a true ministry.
>
> Richard, 33—psychologist

> I was brought up as an atheist but we started going to this progressive Catholic Church while we were still figuring out what was wrong with me and we really felt at home. We realized that we wouldn't be long-term members but the priest talked about things I cared about right then.
>
> Clyde, 39—administrator

> I am a deeply religious person. Once I knew I had this disease, I felt like I gave over to divine guidance and was able to put the future out of my mind. I left the outcome in God's hands.
>
> Robert, 64—professor

Our society suggests that there is an objective reality and you are in it. Buddhism says you can choose the lens you view things through—one way is to view our life with equanimity.

Chris, 51—physician

I asked members of the clergy what people are seeking from their religious leaders at this point. Ron Nofziger, a health-care chaplain in Tulsa, Oklahoma, said, "They want someone who can help them vent and process, someone who can give them answers, like to the 'Why?' question—'Why me? Why my child? What will become of me, of my marriage, of my family, of my job?' This is not really so much a question as it is a lament, a powerful expression of grief. They are sometimes so angry—the whole family is angry, but they think they are forbidden to be angry with God. So I offer them a safe place to vent, to express their anger with God."

He went on: "Rabbi Harold Kushner, after 9/11, said that in moments of deep grief, it is not time to theologize, it is a time to grieve. I think that's what people need: someone who won't take their grief away or trivialize it but someone who will sit with them as a calm, supporting presence. I can't make this disease go away, but if I can provide this, they will be better. Not cured, but better."

Rabbi and psychologist Simkha Weintraub, director of the Center for Jewish Healing in New York City, commented that "People don't know what they are looking for when they call us— kind of whatever is out there—a connection, a path, some way to be normal again. Sometimes people need to tell their story. Some people are curious. The tragedy of medicine now is that the person gets lost. I ignore the time frame the doctor has given them and focus on the person. I want to know who they are and what they are bringing to this challenge of illness."

Appendix F describes some of the key differences among health-care chaplains, pastoral counselors, and clergy that may be relevant if you decide to seek this kind of support.

Talk to Others Facing a Similar Challenge

Some people are eager to hear what it is like to have this condition and go through the various treatments. It helps them anticipate what lies ahead for them to hear about what others have experienced and how they coped. People are not interested in the experiences of others, sometimes because they don't want to hear frightening stories or because they don't have the energy to reach out to anyone new. And then, of course, some people are not the least curious about knowing what someone else has gone through, especially since they are still hoping that they won't have to actually go through any of it themselves.

If you are interested in talking with someone who has your condition or who has undergone the treatment you are considering, there are a number of ways to approach finding them. Your doctor may be willing to refer you to someone he or she has treated who has volunteered to talk to other patients. One of your many friends who told you that they know someone with "exactly your disease" might be willing to ask if that person will talk with you.

> My aunt introduced me to a woman who had had my condition and we hit it off. We didn't do anything formal, just called each other about once a week. It was helpful at the very beginning because I felt like such a novice—I didn't really know how anything about even what questions to ask and she had just a little more experience than I did. I felt less anxious about the side effect and the fatigue.
>
> Aki, 35—receptionist

A number of the national health nonprofit organizations operate telephone services, online discussion lists, and chat rooms staffed by people who have been treated for the disease and who have been trained to talk with newly diagnosed people (see appendix G). You increase the possibility that you will find someone sensitive and knowledgeable by using a service or contacting an organization where the people answering the phone or replying to your e-mail message have some kind of training. Online you may want initially to look for chat rooms or support groups that are moderated by a professional.

> Someone put an organization in touch with me and I kept getting calls from people who were supposed to help me but really, they just wanted to tell me their story. It was good to know there was someone out there,

but they bombarded me and I wasn't really in any shape to listen to them. You can always just say, "Hey! Thanks for talking with me," and hang up if what they are telling you is too upsetting or they are too pushy about what you should do. They are supposed to help you. I did this to one person and their organization called me back a few times. I just ignored them.

Rena, 39—personal trainer

The Internet offers thousands of chat rooms and online discussion lists for various diseases. Some people I talked to tried these immediately after they were diagnosed.

As soon as I was diagnosed, I joined the Listserve [for my disease] and told my story. They were very welcoming and it was great. But I quickly turned into a lurker. It scared me. I'll go on there and skim it or glance at it, but I still don't participate. I feel like I'll go back there when I need to.

Hannah, 37—teacher

Generally, well–established online communities are generous and encouraging to people who are newly diagnosed, but when I recently took a spin through a monitored chat room of a large health voluntary organization, I was surprised to see a preponderance of tough–love ("*Snap out of it! It's only___.*"), competitive ("*You only have X? Well I have Y and that's much worse.*"), and judgmental religious responses ("*It's God's will.*") that drove me shuddering out the door of that electronic room.

Some people I talked with commented that the focus of the discussions of many online support groups that are not specifically for the newly diagnosed tended to be among participants with advanced disease who were advising others whose illnesses were progressing—or about scientific advances that were relevant only to those for whom all other treatments had failed. This information was just not relevant yet—and they hoped it would never be.

Interestingly, most people I talked with who used the Internet returned months later and found the resources online immensely helpful, though they described needing to invest some time in searching for the ones that matched their style and preferences.

Join a Support Group

Online discussion lists and chat rooms offer a middle or even anonymous ground between talking to an individual and joining a support group.

Considerable research has been conducted about the effectiveness of support groups for people who are ill. The evidence shows that such groups are helpful to many people in reducing their distress and helping them to feel better equipped to care for themselves and their condition. However, the majority of this research on the effects of support groups has not looked at their effectiveness for people who are newly diagnosed.

Few people I interviewed were initially attracted to the idea of participating in a formal support group, whether in person or on the telephone. They felt that this was something they might consider later, but that they needed to take care of the medical part of their condition right now. But a few had scouted around to find a group for newly diagnosed people and found immense comfort in the fellowship of the other shocked and dismayed novices.

> When I had the first meeting with the oncologist, I was aware of being alone. I am single and my family lives far away. I knew that I was going to need help to go through it. I asked him if he could recommend a support group and this turned out to be the most important thing for me. I tried two groups: one group that was a stable, long-term commitment group. The other one was for young people with cancer—that helped me—gave me perspective and made me feel less sorry for myself.
>
> But the other one was so unbelievably helpful—both practically and emotionally. It happened to be a group of really thoughtful, caring women, all with bad diagnoses. Seeing that core group every week was so important! We really helped each other.
>
> Nell, 33—lawyer

Mental health professionals I interviewed confirmed what people and their families said about support groups. Margaret Kirk, president of Y–Me, a nonprofit that serves people with breast cancer, noted that "Most people are not attracted to them initially. Many people's first response anyway is 'I don't do groups.' But don't say that until you try: the groups at the Alzheimer's Association are remarkable. It's not just that people understand you—it's that there some of those people are so extraordinarily resourceful and have so much experience that you can't overvalue it."

The availability of support groups for newly diagnosed people seems to depend to some extent on the disease. HIV/AIDS organizations identify this time as particularly important, as do a few cancer groups, and your geographic location may influence the availability and quality of the groups. Veterans of support groups and mental health professionals suggest looking for groups that are led by professionals and whose membership is of people at a similar point post diagnosis.

> I didn't want to meet a whole bunch of new people and hear about what their fears were. I had plenty of fears of my own. Plus I was busy working out what I needed to do next.
>
> Dean, 63—professor

Make Use of Complementary Medicine

About 60 percent of adults in the United States made use of non-conventional therapies in 2004 and a good number of them did so in order to "enhance the mind's capacity to affect physical functions and symptoms and hinge on the body's innate healing capacity" (*Wall Street Journal*, March 15, 2005). So it was no surprise to hear that most people I interviewed had used such methods, including traditional approaches from their family's ethnic or cultural background, to restore their health and spirits. They made creative use of these strategies on the assumption that they wouldn't hurt and might help.

> I took up yoga for relief and my husband and I learned to meditate. We are not religious people and this was so very helpful.
>
> Eleanor, 64—consultant

> I used acupuncture and Chinese herbal medicine. I have found these helpful. I was so depleted and feel like these brought me back.
>
> William, 50—computer programmer

I visited a naturopath and a nutritionist. It's not that I wanted to do anything radical. I just wanted to do everything I could to be healthy so that my body could fight off this disease for as long as it could. What it added in making my life more complicated because it was a whole other set of doctors and substances I had to remember to take, it made up for in me feeling like I was taking care of myself.

Manuel, 62—real estate investor

Consider applying the same standards to finding complementary treatments and practitioners that you have used to find the right medical treatments and specialists. After all, if the complementary therapy is potent enough to make the changes you hope for, why would you view it with more or less caution than you would a standard medical approach just because it is "natural" or "traditional"? You want someone who has a lot of experience treating people who have your condition. Get referrals and references, and talk to the practitioner in person.

Identify what you are trying to achieve with complementary techniques. There are practices that claim to strengthen your immune system, boost your energy, help you relax, or relieve pain. Few of these approaches have been subjected to extensive measurement using scientific methods. Nevertheless, it is a good idea to track down whatever supporting evidence is available.

"If you find a qualified practitioner and you check it with your doctor, try a few treatments—acupuncture, herbs, massage—they work fairly quickly," says Andrew Robinson, a patient advocate. Talking to your doctor can be tough, he notes. "Doctors are more open to acupuncture and massage these days. They don't see any benefit but also anticipate no harm. They get concerned with herbs, though. There is some evidence that they may interact with your medicine."

Robinson advises that physicians have a variety of attitudes toward complementary medicine, not all of them benevolent. You can get information from your practitioner to give to your physician or ask if the practitioner can call and talk about your case. Regardless of your physician's receptiveness, you definitely should let her know what approaches you are using.

Seek Counseling

Bill Breitbart, a psychiatrist at Memorial Sloan-Kettering, used this analogy about seeking counseling after a devastating diagnosis: "Just going through this—all the appointments, all the doctors, all the tests—is like running a marathon. And doing it when you are really upset is like running a marathon with a fifty-pound backpack. I can't make it so you don't have to run the marathon, but I can help lighten the load of that backpack."

Here are four situations for which counseling might be very helpful:

- If you find yourself so upset that you can't think straight, can't rest, can't stop crying, or can't figure out what to do next.

- If you want to talk with someone about the meaning of your life, and you are not religious or your clergyperson isn't able to talk with you about this.

- If you are very frightened about your life, the impending pain of your disease and treatment and the prospect of your death, and you don't have anyone to talk with about this.

- If you are so sad that the burden of your hopelessness makes it difficult for you to get out of bed or make decisions or talk with the people you love.

People often believe they should be able to talk to family and friends about how their diagnosis affects them emotionally but many find it difficult; they don't want to show weakness or let their loved ones down by betraying doubt and fear about the future.

Margo Hover, a health-care chaplain in St. Louis, recounted an encounter with an elderly couple in the hall of the hospital waiting for outpatient chemotherapy. She inquired how they were doing and the husband responded: "She's going to be just fine." His wife looked at him and said, "That's what you keep saying but at night when you are asleep, I realize that I'm dying and you won't let me talk about it."

> I made an appointment with my therapist right away. I knew I needed all the support and reinforcement I could get to go through this. Sometimes it's the only place I can just sit and cry. I can't do that with my husband or in front of my kids and it gets old for my friends.
>
> Georgia, 46—television producer

> My partner and I went to counseling together. The substance of it was how to "metabolize" the seriousness of this illness. We felt like our beautiful life was over. It was important for us to have someone who knew us help us go through this.
>
> Charlotte, 45—professor

Greg, seventy, a retired lawyer, talked about being alone in his hospital room three days after heart surgery:

> This guy comes in and introduces himself. He was really informal and friendly and we talked about the Red Sox and then he says, "You've been through a lot here. How are you doing?" and I burst into tears. Turns out he was the psychiatrist for the surgical unit. He came back another time before I left the hospital and told me that many people got depressed after this operation and told me I could call if I needed to.

Laura Tracy, a psychotherapist who works with seriously ill people in Washington, D.C., explained, "One of the things people who get themselves to a therapist just after a diagnosis want is help calming down and some guidance through treatment options. Not expert medical guidance—more like 'This sounds reasonable' or 'You sound like you really prefer this choice.' Many people find that the first month is about the terror of dying and the fear of pain. The existential crisis seems to come later."

Talking to a professional who has experience with people who are confronting a grave medical condition can be very helpful. Appendix F describes a number of different kinds of mental health professionals you might consider talking with and how to find them.

What about Family Support?

Interesting question. Intuitively, it would seem that family members would provide the kind of familiar and unconditional love that would be most likely to provide relief during this time. But when asked about what worked to give them a break from their distress, the people I interviewed did not mention their families.

This is not to say that people did not talk about their families and those closest to them. Many people described about how their families reacted, supported, and failed to support members who had just received a serious diagnosis. And it is not to say that people were not grateful for the shelter and warmth provided by their children and parents and siblings and spouses and partners. They don't know how they would have gotten through this period without them, but few identify family members as instrumental in providing relief.

Perhaps this is because if you are close enough to be considered a "loved one," you are close enough to feel the same sense of crisis and impending loss, and thus are in similar need of some moments in which to recharge your batteries.

Or, perhaps, you are so wrapped up in the unfolding drama together—you share every piece of information, your conversations are riveted on the subject of the diagnosis, the meaning of this diagnosis is catastrophic for both of you—that it is only through retiring to separate corners that you can find a moment to regroup.

Or maybe long-standing conflicts and ways of interacting that have caused friction in the past are heightened by the intensity of this crisis.

This can be such a lonely time for couples and families! So much talking goes on, yet so much is unsaid.

> I lied to my wife about how I felt. I didn't want her to think that all she was doing for me was for naught. And she lied to me. She was cheerful and upbeat. She didn't want me to know how frightened she was because she thought I would be discouraged and unwilling to go on.
>
> David, 64—environmentalist

One woman said her husband, an accountant, was so determined to keep his illness a secret he was unwilling to allow her even to call the nurse to inquire about symptoms following a test. "I couldn't do anything without him knowing. I had him for support, but I couldn't tell friends. Sometimes I would go for a walk and call my daughter on the cell phone and just vent. The kids were a wonderful support but I didn't want to burden them."

During these first days following a devastating diagnosis, everyone is still getting their feet back under them. Families and couples haven't yet figured out how they are going to manage this crisis and as they thrash about, they sometimes say and do things that are damaging or disappointing. The intensity of emotions and sense of emergency heightens everyone's sense of danger, of urgency. Everyone needs a little relief, a little time out from thinking about this problem and from each other.

CHAPTER 10

Take Your Next Steps

Your aim is to make decisions that you are confident are right for you and that will allow you to live as well and as long as you can.

Getting a devastating diagnosis is like being pushed into a rushing river. You paddle madly to stay afloat as you are carried along by the unfolding disease and what it means. Every once in a while you need to fight your way to the side of the river to catch your breath. What is this experience like? How are you doing? Can you take a little break and think about what you need and want?

—Bruce Doblin, internist and hospice physician, Chicago

COME ON OVER TO THE EDGE of the river out of the current and rest for a minute.

Take a few deep breaths.

What do you need right now? What is going to help you move forward, to feel like you are making progress? Do you need to make a decision about medical treatment—which one to have—or whether to get treated at all? Do you need to make some choices about how to manage your condition—now and over time?

Many people manage to plan to respond to their diagnosis within a month or six weeks after getting the first bad news. They know what is coming next: some kind of treatment—surgery, drugs—or a period of waiting for the disease or its symptoms to develop or not. And they have arranged their lives to begin to accommodate the demands of the disease and its treatment. They breathe a sigh of relief and launch themselves into the next phase.

Getting to this point is not simple. The language and logic of medicine are linear, and life—especially now—is not like that. Rather, it is at the mercy of doctors' availability, the results of a new test, or the emergence of a new symptom. Of course, part of moving forward means making decisions about how to respond medically to your diagnosis.

But the actual treatment choice affects and is affected by your own unique web of circumstances: your family situation, financial status, personal relationships, interests and preferences, physical and emotional energy, and work arrangements.

Occasionally, people talk with their doctor and family members, and make quick decisions about treatment and care. Many of us, however, for a variety of reasons, find ourselves getting stuck along the way. It may be that our physicians are too busy to talk with us about treatment options and their implications, or we find ourselves faced with making treatment decisions that are too technical for us to feel comfortable with. It may be that the complications of work and family and other responsibilities feel overwhelming. We may be too frightened to make a choice from which there is no road back. Or maybe we are just too tired to make one more decision.

This chapter begins with planning. It describes considerations about making treatment decisions, then it discusses some of the places people I talked to got stuck—where unexpected entanglements kept them from moving forward.

The next section will help you think about what kind of help you might seek as you and your family adjust to the emerging demands of your condition and its treatment.

The chapter ends with some reflections about taking the next steps by both me and those I interviewed for this book: What it is like to leave behind this high-anxiety, high-pressure period of shock, and to head into the different—but no less engrossing—phase during which you pull together your resources and hopes and sail into the next part of your life.

Want to Make God Laugh? Tell Him Your Plan

I initially thought this chapter would be called "Make Your Plan" because theoretically, that's what you do. You gather all this information and then, after consulting with doctors, friends, and family, you decide how you are going to head this condition off.

You will think through medical or other measures intended

to cure it or slow its course and perhaps through personal actions that will strengthen your resistance and amplify the effects of the medical care.

But this is just theory. All the people I interviewed with bad diagnoses and their loved ones reminded me of my own experience with life-altering diagnoses.

We don't make a plan to respond to the diagnosis. Rather, we figure out what we are going to try first, and if that doesn't work, we try the next thing. And if that doesn't work, we try again. And again. We do this with our treatment and we do this as we adjust to the demands of the condition on our lives. I try working and it becomes too complicated, I take a leave of absence. You keep going to the poker game and beg off when it becomes more of a burden than a pleasure.

This is where we come squarely up against the uncertainty that characterizes medicine in the twenty-first century. While developments in diagnosis and treatment have been amazing in recent decades, so much remains unknown!

Sometimes we are seduced into believing that the clean statistics that are used to quantify our blood, our brain functions, our kidney output, and the size and type of our tumors mean that there are equally clean, calibrated treatments that can fix what's wrong. If the process of getting your diagnosis confirmed and identifying your treatment options haven't convinced you that this is not the case, taking the next steps will.

So what, really, does it mean to decide to take the next steps? Let's start with treatment.

For some people with some conditions, the first course of action is clear: the evidence-based standard care, tailored to fit your personal characteristics, is the starting point. You get those polyps surgically removed and start a regimen of chemotherapy. You initiate the standard course of antiretroviral drugs to control HIV. Or you investigate all the vision aids that are available to help you maintain your livelihood as you lose your sight.

But for many, the confirmed diagnosis of a life-altering condition doesn't trigger an automatic first step. The diagnosis is the end of one kind of uncertainty but the beginning of another. Do you start interferon as soon as relapsing-remitting MS is diagnosed or do you wait? Do you wait for symptoms of leukemia to emerge before you start chemotherapy? Which drug do you try first to delay

Parkinson's symptoms? Do you choose a mastectomy or lumpectomy; prostatectomy or radiation plus chemotherapy?

Or do you want medical intervention at all? You may be
leaning toward an alternative, whether that means refusing treatment because you are fatalistic and you think "your number is
up"; your faith leads you to decline medical intervention; you
believe your body will naturally heal itself; or you choose to use
alternative medicine approaches to treat your disease.

For a number of people I interviewed, the question of whether
to make use of medical interventions was on the table from the
moment they were diagnosed. Most ultimately chose to make use
of the tools of medicine, even if selectively, for example, to ease
their pain.

> I made the decision to try nonmedical approaches to healing my early
> breast cancer for quite a while. It was not what my doctor recom-
> mended, but there was a much bigger chance that it would not metas-
> tasize than that it would and I took a risk that I would be one of the
> lucky ones. Eventually I had to have a mastectomy.
>
> Rena, 39—personal trainer

For all of those who considered alternatives to medical treatment,
as well as all of those who were faced with a choice about what
treatment to pursue, the decisions were rarely simple.

How Do I Make Decisions about Treatment?

I was absolutely stuck for a month about whether I should have
surgery or should "watchfully wait" to see how fast the cancer
that was left in me after the biopsy was growing. On one hand
there was the prospect of a hysterectomy and thus the loss
of my ability to have children and on the other, the torturous
anxiety about whether the doctors would detect the enemy
within in time to save me—a fear heightened by too vivid and
too recent memories of being ravaged by the surgery, endless
radiation, and years of chemotherapy of my previous cancer diagnosis.

At any given time, I was completely convinced that one of
these choices was the only one that made sense. The problem was

that if you asked me an hour later, I would be equally convinced that the other option was the right one.

Did I ask for help when I was making up my mind? You bet. But everyone I approached, including all my doctors, said that only I could make this decision because only I knew whether I, over time, could tolerate the anxiety of a recurrence or be willing to forgo bearing children. Even the trick of asking the doctors what they would advise their daughters to do couldn't smoke out guidance.

I eventually wore myself down. I couldn't bear to think about it anymore and I decided—somewhat arbitrarily, ultimately—that I would eventually adjust to either decision. I scheduled the surgery. I felt relieved. I started to think about how my life would be different.

I felt very alone in making this decision. It was as though people thought that if they talked about the pros and cons of my choices with me—or even asked me what I was thinking about choosing—that they would be making my decision for me.

Of course, for many health conditions there is a clearly preferred treatment. Bacterial pneumonia is always treated with antibiotics, for example, and is almost always cured. "In primary care, probably ninety percent of what goes on is fairly straightforward. But in most specialties—like mine—hematology and oncology—most decisions are not clear-cut," says Dr. Jerome Groopman, a professor at Harvard Medical School whose popular books and articles help patients navigate the complications of twenty-first-century medicine. "Often, strong evidence is lacking or there is not consensus about what works."

So how do doctors decide which treatment is right for a particular patient? David Nathan, an oncologist and former president of the Dana Farber Cancer Institute at Harvard Medical School, says, "In the moment of decision, a physician must be guided but not dominated by evidence-based medicine [the results of clinical trials]. Instead she must weigh the likelihood of success for an *individual* patient against what she believes is the tolerance of the patient for the treatment under consideration. Clinical trials are averages, and they may be difficult to reproduce. In the end, it is quality of life for a *particular* patient that matters."

And because there are now more options for treatments, all of which we hope will affect the course of our disease and may influence the quality of our lives, there is growing attention to the role of patients in making decisions about care and treatment. That said, despite the rise in health-care consumerism, some physicians are still not comfortable coaching patients to examine the pros and cons of each option, and many patients prefer their doctor to make a firm recommendation.

However, if the interviews for this book are any indication—and that includes people with serious diseases as well as health professionals of all stripes—there is a rising expectation that an individual's preferences and values will be included in some treatment decisions.

Specifically, you may be asked to make choices about treatments when*:

- *There are major differences in the types of outcomes the different treatments offer.* For example, imminent death versus severe disability.

- *There are major differences between the treatments in the likelihood and impact of complications.* For example, one treatment may not be very effective but it has few side effects, whereas the alternative treatment is probably more effective but the chances of having severe, permanent effect on your ability to function are greater.

- *Your choices involve trade-offs between near-term and long-term outcomes.* For example, one treatment may offer a few more months of vision but will result in certain blindness, whereas the other offers an uncertain decline in sight over time.

- *One of the choices carries a small risk of a grave outcome.* For example, one out of 100,000 people who get this operation die from it.

- *The apparent difference between options is marginal.* For example, in some cases of breast cancer, treatment with a lumpectomy or mastectomy do not differ in the outcomes predicted over time.

*Adapted from J. Kassirer, "Incorporating Patients' Preferences into Medical Decisions," *New England Journal of Medicine* 330, no. 26 (June 30, 1994): 1895–96.

- *You are genuinely averse to taking risks.* For example, you only want treatments that have been determined to be safe, even if there may be others that are still experimental but might be more effective.

- *You attach special importance to certain possible outcomes.* For example, under no circumstances do you want to be dependent on a ventilator.

- *There is a hint of an answer on the research horizon but it's not there yet.* You might have read of some early-stage animal research that looks promising but results for humans are years away. [I added this item to Kassirer's list based on my experiences and those of the people I interviewed.]

A doctor can describe your treatment options, can talk about the chances of producing a given outcome and can provide details about the side effects that have been observed in others. But only one person can imagine what each choice would mean to *you*.

Here are the pieces of the puzzle that will help you make a decision in which you have confidence:

- *You need to know about your choices.* What would the different medical treatments consist of? What are the likely results of each one? What are the side effects now and over time? What would happen if you decided not to make use of *any* medical treatment? See chapter 5 for a list of questions to ask your doctor and appendix A for resources that can help you answer them.

- *You need to think about and decide which outcomes matter to you most.* Bruce Doblin, a primary care physician in Chicago who has played an active role with many of his patients after a devastating diagnosis, says that he asks patients, "What is it that you really want? What is important to you? What are your goals? What would you work the hardest to preserve?"

- *You need to think through what is important to you in achieving these outcomes.* As noted in chapter 5, you will want to consider practical factors, for example, "Can I afford this treatment?" Your choice will also be influenced by your preferences: for example, "I do not want to live with the anxiety of doing nothing about this disease." And your values will play a powerful role, for example, "My mind is me: I don't want to be so out of it with pain medication that I can't think."

- *You need to be able to make your values and preferences clear to your doctor so that he or she can tailor your treatment to them as much as possible.* This should not be too much to ask of your doctor, said Jerome Groopman. "You need a physician who first speaks to you as an individual and demonstrates that he or she has heard you and has considered the specifics of your situation, whether they are clinical, social, emotional, religious, occupational—whatever is important to you.

   "For many of these decisions, there is a prototype of the patient this treatment works for. But no patient fits the prototype. There is benefit in having evidence—but the decisions produced from this discussion are the art of medicine. Otherwise everything could be done by computer—you wouldn't need doctors."

   "Doctors talk about facts and probabilities—the probability of benefit, harm, and side effects," says Annette O'Connor, a researcher at the University of Ottawa, who has investigated how people make these types of decisions. "Patients talk about values—and the impact different options would have on their life. Both need to hear what the other is saying."

The tough thing is to not make this decision on the fly. You have so much to do; you are finding out new information every day; the picture goes in and out of focus; it is not exactly clear what you are deciding between or whether you have any choices at all.

Looking back on the times when I had to make such decisions, it is a little hard for me to see why I didn't take the time to think these decisions through in an orderly way. I seemed to be attracted to the deeply uncomfortable decide-in-a-panic-in-the-middle-of-the-night approach. Every night, I obsessed about my choices as I tossed and turned. As soon as I thought I had made my decision and was falling asleep, I would realize that I had forgotten about a whole set of possible side effects that I feared, or would remember how long one treatment lasted versus the other and the whole thing would start up again.

And it's not as though I don't know that I think more clearly in the daylight and that decisions seem more manageable when I write my thoughts down and talk about them with others. But somehow, it was always hard for me to find the time.

Perhaps you'll do better. This doesn't have to be that hard.

If you have to make a decision, see if you can't take a half hour to sit down with someone you trust and talk the decision through, writing out the pros and cons of each choice as described above, making sure you really are considering what it is you want and what each of your treatment choices—perhaps including the no-treatment option—offers you.

If you need some structure for doing this, see if your health plan offers guidance in making such decisions through its advice line or coaching program, or on the plan's Web site. If not, take a look at the free sources of decision support noted in appendix A.

"People really resist using these pen-and-paper and online decision aids—my own mom thought it was stupid. But I sat with her and we did it together. In hindsight, most people find that they learned things and that it made them more confident that they were making the right decision for themselves," says Annette O'Connor.

The purpose of using decision support of any kind is to prepare for your discussion with your physician about treatment. By doing so, you will also be able to identify gaps in your knowledge and think about your own values and needs and preferences.

Once you and your doctor have come to a decision, ask her to lay out what will happen next—what treatments you need to get, what tests, at what intervals. Find out how and under what circumstances you will communicate with one another, what symptoms and side effects you should look out for, how you will know if this course of action is working, and what her plan is in the event that it is not. You need this information to move forward with confidence.

What Do You Need to Be Able to Function?

Psychiatric clinical nurse specialist Janet Baradell often talks with families as they adjust to a new serious diagnosis of one of their members. She told me that she finds that, just after a diagnosis of a serious condition, many people sit on their emotions until things are really settled. She noted that they are much more likely to want to solve the problems of daily functioning: Who will care for my kids while I am in the hospital? How will I manage if I can no longer drive? Who will take care of my disabled husband while I am in cardiac rehab?

True? Probably. But not always.

If you are too distressed to start this problem-solving—or are too sad—or if you find yourself getting really angry really easily so that it is damaging your relationships with those you love, consider looking for some help. Chapter 9 offers different approaches to finding relief and appendix F describes a number of sources of professional support.

But the day-to-day management challenges of a serious illness still have to be overcome. Here are some of the places where the people I interviewed described getting stuck and a description of the help they sought in order to move on.

Don't get me wrong here. I am not suggesting that you surround yourself with professionals who will be able to carry you through this time unscathed. As you know, what you are experiencing can't be delegated or outsourced to South Asia. But I know how easy it is to feel bewildered by all the new information and demands, and there are many resources that you might not think of or know about.

Say I am still not ready to make the big decisions about my care. Who, besides my specialists and my family, can I talk with who will help me think about what is right for me?

When I talked to people about how they made these life-altering decisions about treatment under stress, some said they needed to talk through the decision with a medical professional who didn't have a stake in which choice they made, while others just wanted to talk it through with someone who they trusted to listen and not judge them.

My take-home advice to anyone going through this is to find a good primary care provider—a family doctor or an advanced practice nurse and involve them in your decision and then in your care after that. No one else is going to pay attention to your side effects and symptoms and notice when you are depressed. No one else is going to look at how your condition is affecting your family—it won't even come up. The specialists are busy focusing on your disease, not on you.

Chuck, 45—teacher

About five years ago I asked a friend of mine if he would be willing to talk with me about raising my kids. He's a retired cop, actually—who I think is smart and wise and has been a good father and husband. I lost my father when I was pretty young and I thought he would be a good one to talk to when my daughters hit adolescence. Anyway, it turned out that he was the best person for me to talk with about making this decision.

Jed, 43—state health official

I was really under the gun to make a decision about my treatment—six weeks had gone by and I was getting a lot of pressure from my doctors and my parents. They each had a different idea about what I should do. Finally I made an appointment to see a psychotherapist. I felt safe talking with her. She didn't have a vested interest. I felt that my words had weight. I wasn't just a body on the assembly line they were bending to their will.

Nell, 33—lawyer

How can I get a handle on what is going on when it seems like no one is in charge and I have five doctors all weighing in with their way of treating my condition?

This can happen whether you are inside the hospital or outside if your condition is complicated or rare or very fragile or if you have received a number of conflicting opinions about what treatment will give you the best outcome.

Psychologist Ken Gorfinkle recounted how a distraught woman approached him in the hall of the hospital and said, "Doctors keep coming in and out of my husband's room. Each one looks at the chart and orders different tests and none of them seem to read what the others have ordered. I think some of these tests are being repeated. Don't they talk to each other? Who is in charge?"

And his response was that, unfortunately, it looked like she was.

It places an extraordinary burden on a patient or family member to assume the role of executive manager of experts and to learn how to coordinate complex institutional arrangements when he or she is gravely ill or in crisis. Yet it happens frequently.

Here are some ways people responded to this situation:

When my wife was very ill with breast cancer, we just let the doctors duke it out among themselves and it was a mess. But in the aftermath of my (adult) daughter's brain tumor, we hired a quarterback, very senior neurologist, expressly for the purpose of talking to all the doctors and then meeting with my daughter about once a month to see how she's doing and discuss the options. It's not great but it is less confusing.

Harry, 78—retired advertising executive

After a lot of trial and error and confusion, a lot of annoyance among family members, and a couple of blow-ups with this one doctor in the hospital, we finally designated one person—my son—to be the point person with all the doctors. He wasn't intimidated by them and he is pretty even-tempered. He did a good job of getting them to write things down so he could make sure all of them had all the same information.

Nora, 78—homemaker

We reached a crisis when they hospitalized my mother to do a procedure she didn't understand or want done. There was too much of this—doctors who wanted to do procedures that were marginally indicated and who didn't think they needed to explain things to me or to my mom. I fired them all when I found a family practice doctor, a geriatrician who was willing to come in and get to the bottom of what needed to be done. Afterward, this family doctor coordinated my mother's care—and called in specialists when they were needed. She works with a nurse practitioner and the resident who went to visit my mom regularly. She would call a meeting with my mom and all her doctors and nurses when I came to town.

Emily, 60—social worker

My health plan has a health coaching service. I called them to get advice about how to handle this problem of all these specialists taking care of my husband and no one was taking the lead. They couldn't do anything about the doctors but it helped to talk it through and get some perspective. Afterward I felt like I was more organized and able to ask better questions.

Terry, 36—foundation executive

Who can help me figure out how to make the transition from what was *to* what is now—*like how to bring my husband home after his stroke or how to recover from bypass surgery?*

Depending on your diagnosis, you may need to make significant changes in the way you live if you (or if the person who is sick) is going to live at home. Whether the changes are immediate (if your partner has had a stroke and can't walk or feed herself, for example)—or gradual over time (for example, if you have a progressive neuromuscular condition), there is a maze of services and benefits for which you might be eligible. Much is known about the practical aspects of adapting to a variety of physical and cognitive limitations:

I am a nurse and I swear by the medical social worker who helped me when I was getting ready to leave the hospital after I had my leg amputated. She knew everything that was available in our town, she knew what insurance would cover and how to get it covered, she knew what I needed—I couldn't believe it. She was invaluable at a time when I was not thinking clearly.

Judy, 66—nurse

The Alzheimer's Association has really useful information on the Web site about taking care of people with Alzheimer's disease at home—you know, how to keep a routine, how to organize the house, what to expect, the importance of respite care. Plus there is a phone number [1-800-272-3900] you call to say "I'm having this problem," and people with lots of experience and training will give you practical suggestions.

Hope, 69—archivist

Just before my husband came home from the hospital after his stroke we had a conversation with a clinical nurse specialist about me now becoming the caregiver. She said, "Just because you are the wife and can physically provide the care doesn't mean that you have to do all of it." What a relief! The three of us had a conversation about needs and expectations and responsibilities. She helped us find some services and get some benefits we didn't even know existed. She also referred us to the National Family Caregivers—they have a Web site and phone number and they have been a great resource for me.

Maria, 74—matriarch

I keep coming up with new questions: Is this symptom related to my condition? Is my stomach upset due to my medication? Should I be taking vitamins? Should I consider doing this new treatment I just heard about on the news? Why am I so tired? I feel like someone should have told me this stuff. I don't want to bother my specialist with all these questions but I sure would like some answers.

Cosmically, this is the right time to be asking questions about health, given the incredible resources available—the millions of Web sites, newspaper articles, radio spots, and TV news segments that examine each aspect of the topic.

On the other hand, you probably have questions that are pretty specific to your current situation, what you are experiencing and what to expect. And the kind of personalized information you want may not be easy to find from the generally available sources.

I had so many questions when I was first diagnosed and then again when I started treatment. I happened on the National Cancer Institute telephone help line [1-800-4-cancer]. The people who answer the phone were fabulous. They really knew what they were talking about. I don't know what I would have done without them.

Gara, 53—athletic facility manager

At first I hated to call my doctor with questions because I didn't want to bother her with things that might be routine—but they just weren't routine for me yet. Pretty quickly I learned to call to talk to the nurses in her practice. They were very helpful. They have talked to hundreds of people dealing with the same problems. They know what is weird and what is normal. They know which problems the doctor needs to know about. Plus they are available.

Carmen, 37—hospital clerk

I have had a pretty bad attitude about my health plan—you know, that they just want to save money at my expense. But I called the telephone number that was listed on the plan brochure and the person was able to answer my questions and sent me some things by mail. The person the next time I called wasn't as good, but I'd call again. You don't have to wait for a call back from a doctor or take time off from work to go see one to find out the little stuff you need to know.

Marilyn, 59—minister

What can I do about all this uncertainty about the future?

Receiving a devastating diagnosis increases exponentially the amount of uncertainty you live with day in and day out. Most people I talked to were at first bowled over by having so many of their expectations and assumptions washed away in one brief conversation with a physician.

He took our lives and smashed them on the floor in ten minutes,

Sasha, 62—artist

You can't do much about some of the sources of uncertainty: you simply don't know how your body and the disease and the treatment will interact. But there are parts of the uncertainty that may cause you less anxiety if you give them some attention.

Most people began to regain a foothold when they were able to identify and talk about the specific implications of the diagnosis on their life and the lives of their loved ones.

Asking your doctor to lay out your treatment plan, your respective responsibilities, and his contingency plan in case events don't unfold as expected can help you feel more certain of the immediate future.

As a former nurse, I was trained to look at the worst-case scenario and plan for that. So I always wanted to hear the real statistics. Plus, I had to think ahead: we had my eighty-five-year-old mom with dementia and my daughter and her newborn living with us.

We did this, then, with everything: What if I lost my income? What if we couldn't afford the mortgage? What if? What if? We ran the numbers. We wanted to know and to work it through. The free-floating anxiety was much worse than the worst-case scenario. It was very important during those first couple of weeks to put our financial house in order. We did medical powers of attorney, living wills, regular wills. Then I felt like I could go ahead and take care of this disease.

Eleanor, 64—consultant

My mom, her primary care doctor, and I sat around a table and talked about what kind of care my mother wanted at the end of her life. I didn't know how to talk with her about this or how to help her make these decisions. On the form was the question about whether she should be sent to the hospital or be treated for pneumonia and have a feeding tube. If we hadn't had this conversation beforehand, I don't know how I would have held up under making those decisions.

Emily, 60—social worker

Thoughts on How to Keep Moving

I asked the people I interviewed to reflect on their experience during this time: Were there ideas that were important or lessons they learned that they wanted to pass on? Interestingly, most people declined to offer advice to others going through the early days of a difficult diagnosis, other than to say things like "taking someone else to your appointments with you is pretty darned important!"

Each person I interviewed took the time to talk in detail about painful memories in the hopes that their experience might lessen the burden of someone else going through a similar situation, so, the lack of straightforward advice seemed to be real reticence about generalizing from an experience that was unique to them. As Marilyn, a retired high school teacher, said, "It's a little early to feel that I have transcended this experience and understand its meaning to my life." Lee, a forty-two-year-old architect, said, "Telling someone they would do a lot better if they could feel more hopeful about their situation in the weeks just after they are diagnosed is like telling them that they could probably play for the NBA if they were a lot taller."

Going back through the interviews, however, I found that many people mentioned how they approached taking the next steps.

My husband and I have only talked a couple of times about going to the "dark side." We have each gone there alone. At the beginning I couldn't stop crying—I didn't know how I would be able to function. Someone said, "You have to go to that other side—go somewhere and walk yourself through him dying and you living without him." This was important. It is the fear of the unknown that paralyzes. You can acknowledge the possibilities and know where you might go. It doesn't mean that you are fatalistic and it doesn't mean that it's going to happen.

Georgia, 46—producer

When I was ten, I thought that if one of my parents died, how would I wake up in the morning? How could I go to the funeral of a parent? By coincidence, my mom died a couple of years later and I realize, you just do it—one foot in front of the other. It makes you see that there is so much you can do if the situation requires it.

Harper, 42—teacher

Both my parents are doctors and I had a belief—a fantasy—that medicine was a certain science. One of the things I found hardest was that medicine couldn't give me answers. I could do a lot of research but in the end, it is a leap into the dark.

Nell, 33—lawyer

I never stopped listening to my own sixth sense and I never allowed anyone to dictate to me what they thought I should do with my cancer. No matter who you are or who you have been, you need to understand that you and you alone are the navigator of your treatment. Please welcome people to support you, but never allow them to tell you how to think or feel. You are the only keeper of your heart and mind.

Maral, 44—writer

Reflections on Taking the Next Steps

When I set out to write this book, I thought I would talk to a few people, consult with some thoughtful experts, cast about for a while on the Web and put it all together. I was certain that my own numerous experiences with serious illness and my professional training had prepared me well to organize the material. But I was wrong.

After talking with the first three people about what they thought one ought to know about how to respond to a serious diagnosis, I realized that I had taken too narrow a view of the demands such news places on those of us who are sick and the people who care for us. So I sought out more people who would tell me about their experiences: rich ones, poor ones; people who went through this alone by choice, and those who were alone through circumstance. I found people with insurance and those without, people in big cities and tiny communities, people born in the United States and born elsewhere. I interviewed people who had lived with their disease for years and those who have died since they spoke with me.

Their experiences are described in the previous chapters. The brief glimpses of how individuals approached getting through this time are meant to illustrate for you the many different ways people make use of the maps and compasses of scientific evidence to guide them as they navigate the foreign terrain of serious illness.

But in these descriptions, I am unable to do justice to the energy and focus each person brought to the tasks before them. Each story was unique. Each person solved the problems their disease created in ways that, while rarely ideal, often employed a raw creativity that shone with the stubborn will to live.

Reading over the transcripts of these interviews one last time, I am stuck by what a messy time in a person's life this is. It is a crisis, and your normal life is knocked off-kilter. Information comes in fits and starts, with its meaning and implications trailing behind. We are at the mercy of other people's schedules, of institutional procedures, by medical norms and practices we've never heard of.

I was talking with oncologist Paul Wallace about how he handled information and decision-making with patients. I remarked on how many people I had talked with had felt abandoned by their doctors in this time immediately after a devastating diagnosis, and he said, "The thing that really amazes me is how consistently people are able to move on and do okay, despite our naïve and clumsy efforts."

He is right. The promise of a return to health after a devastating diagnosis lies partly with doctors and hospitals and the medical armamentarium that scientists have developed over the years. It also depends in part on the millions of information Web sites and thousands of support groups, decision aids, books, and pamphlets that are available to help people approach medical care with a basic understanding of their options.

But it was clear to me in listening to people with serious diagnoses and their loved ones that this promise relies most heavily on the responsiveness, the resilience, and the resourcefulness of individuals to get what they need—the promise of returning to a reasonable life relies on the ongoing search for a way to live out your days without pain—to get up every morning and take those drugs that make you feel so tired and stupid; to be willing to try new approaches on the off-chance that they might be effective; and sometimes to say "no more."

So while this is an untidy time and we are confused and impatient participants in this imperfect process, it is in part, our demands and our dreams of what is possible that drive the care we receive.

I was also struck, in rereading more than two hundred interviews, that no matter how much you would like to be able to put all that emotional distress—your own and that of those you love—in a big box and seal it up, in the end, this is impossible to do.

Making rational decisions about doctors and hospitals and treatments and work and family is hard enough without having to confront the fact that the length and quality of your life may hang in the balance of each one. And so it is no surprise that we are brought up short when our will and discipline and competence reach their limits.

It is an illusion, after all, to think that if only we can find the right doctors and get the right treatments and talk with the right professionals, our disease will be checked and we will return to life as it was just a few weeks ago.

Many of us have profound faith in our management skills. We are well connected; we know who to call and how to get things done. We know people who know people. Most of us feel we are fairly effective in our dealings in the world, and we have confidence that we can provide for and protect ourselves and those we love.

Before we received our devastating diagnoses, we tended to get through our days believing that we pretty much knew what was going on and what was going to happen next—and that if something went wrong, there would be some way to fix it or adjust to it. And on occasion, we were jarred out of our sense that the world was an ordered place—an airplane falling out of the sky, the accidental death of a child, the devastation of a hurricane. Such events reminded us of the randomness of fortune and the grand indifference of nature.

A serious diagnosis of disease—our own or that of someone we love—immerses us in that cold, uncomfortable reality. Our connections, our skills in finding information and acting on it, our abilities to cope, all of which are necessary for making the right decisions and getting the right care for us, may not be sufficient to return us whole to the life we had before.

A devastating diagnosis not only challenges our sense of ourselves as stars in the show of our lives but it also rips away our sense that we are somehow in control. Many of us feel that our lives are diminished—that they consist now only of *this* disease, *this* treatment, *this* fatigue, *this* pain.

It is a profound loss that reverberates long after we actually receive the news of our condition.

And so in the midst of the confusion caused by the shock of your diagnosis, it is hard to hold on to the sense that you are more than your disease. You are a participant in a life that is rich with relationships and obligations and possibilities. Your life has been profoundly changed by the diagnosis of the disease.

But you are the same person. Your history, your experiences— all the things that brought you here—remain.

Your aim is to take steps—some big, some small—that build on the certainties you now possess and that will carry you through the unknowable future with all the grace you can muster, all the support you can find, and all the dignity you deserve.

Digging Deeper:
A Guide to Greater Expertise

B Y NOW YOU HAVE PROBABLY DECIDED which kind of person you are when it comes to seeking information about your diagnosis. If you think you come down on the side of the "blunters"—the less detail, the better—there are still a few places out there in the world of health information that might prove useful for you. Of course, if you're a "monitor," on the prowl for each little detail and update about your condition, there are numerous information sources for you to explore.

For everyone, the trick is separating the wheat from the chaff. This appendix provides information search strategies for confirmed blunters and monitors, as well as people who might find both of these strategies useful at different times.

What If I Only Want the Basics?

INTERNET RESOURCES
For people in search of a quick rundown of their condition, the National Institutes of Health (http://health.nih.gov/) Web site might be the best place to start your search. The National Institutes of Health (NIH) is the federal government's premier health research agency. Its general health information Web site allows you to search for information on your condition by its location in the body, the disease name, or health issues such as drug abuse. NIH's health main page also contains links to several other sites mentioned below.

NIH's MedlinePlus (www.nlm.nih.gov/medlineplus/) is also a good one-stop-shopping destination for basic health information. A service of the National Institutes of Health and the U.S. National Library of Medicine, the site contains general information on more than seven hundred diseases and health topics, a medical encyclopedia, information about prescription and over-the-counter medications, a page of links to directories for doctors and hospitals across the country, and information about public medical libraries in your area. The site also contains a collection of short Web movies about certain diseases. Some of the information on the site is available in Spanish.

Finally, WebMD/Medscape (www.webmd.com/) can give you much of the same general information as the two government Web sites just mentioned, but its style may be more friendly to Web surfers who normally don't browse "official-type" sites. One of the original comprehensive sites for health information on the Web, WebMD includes general information on diseases, treatments, and healthy living. The site has a special "newly diagnosed" section that provides a quick introduction to your particular disease and ten questions to ask your doctor on your next visit. WebMD also has a physician search page, and numerous message boards and live chats with medical experts.

Medscape, a decade-old Web database that is now part of the WebMD site, provides more technical information on new research in medical journals.

OVER THE PHONE

The National Institutes of Health offers much of the basic information available on their Web sites through toll-free hotlines. If you do not have access to the Internet, the hotline operators can mail information from specific Web sites, such as the National Cancer Institute, and NIH pamphlets on disease, treatments, and clinical trials. NIH will send up to twenty publications free of charge, and as many publications as you like after that for the cost of shipping. Operators can also search for clinical trials in your area. Many hotlines also feature prerecorded information about a disease. The hotline information is also available in Spanish.

Some of the major NIH hotlines include:

HIV/AIDS: 1 (800) HIV-0440

Alzheimer's Disease: 1 (800) 438-4380

Cancer: 1 (800) 4-CANCER

Heart, Lung, and Blood Disease: 1 (800) 575-WELL

Diabetes: 1 (800) 860–8747

Brain, Spinal Cord, and Nerve Diseases: 1 (800) 352–9424

Stroke: 1 (800) 352–9424

A full list of the hotlines is available at: http://healthhotlines .nlm.nih.gov/index.html.

That's a Good Start, but I Need to Know More

If you have checked out the resources above and still feel you need to find more detailed information or different ways of learning about your condition, there are many other resources available for further exploration. Most of the resources listed below are Web sites, but these resources often have hotlines or other ways besides the Internet to get their information.

Thanks, that's enough information for me.
But now how do I make sense of it?

If these sources of general information about your condition seem to contain everything you want to know at this point, you still need to make sense of what you read or hear. The two Web resources below can be very useful at this stage of your search. You can use their tips for identifying accurate and unbiased scientific information.

MedlinePlus: Evaluating Health Information (www.nlm .nih.gov/medlineplus/evaluatinghealthinformation.html) is an excellent clearinghouse from NIH's MedlinePlus. This page contains links to a number of articles that can help you understand what makes a good scientific study, how to find reliable health information on the Internet, and how to track down specific information about your condition.

Deciphering Medspeak (www.mlanet.org/resources/medspeak/index.html) This site from the Medical Library Association contains a very simple glossary that translates medical terms into everyday language and a guide to the confusing medical shorthand that your doctors may use on your prescriptions, along with more resources on evaluating health Web sites.

I need more information about my specific condition.

Some of the best sources for information about specific conditions are voluntary nonprofit organizations that are disease specific, such as the American Cancer Society. These organizations can give you general information about your condition, treatment, and quality of life. They can also direct you to local resources, such as support groups and clinics that specialize in your condition. These organizations are also a good source of up-to-date information on new drugs, clinical trials, and scientific findings related to a particular disease.

For more information on the services offered by some of the larger organizations, check out "Voluntary Nonprofit Organizations" (appendix G) on page 242.

If you have health insurance, your health plan may offer information on particular conditions on its Web site or in pamphlets that you can request from the company. Although the information may overlap with what you read on larger sites such as WebMD, it may include specific information on the treatments covered by the plan or physicians within the plan that specialize in your condition. Some of the larger, national insurers have extensive health information sites:

Blue Cross Blue Shield
www.bcbs.com/resources/index.html

Aetna
www.intelihealth.com/IH/ihtIH?r=WSAUS000

Kaiser Permanente
www.kaiserpermanente.org/

Other sources of disease-specific information include:

American Academy of Family Physicians
http://familydoctor.org/
This general health Web site allows users to search for information on specific symptoms. The site also contains a Web

review page, updated monthly, that highlights useful and accurate sites for specific conditions.

Medem for Patients
http://medem.com/pat/pat.cfm
Medem provides e-mail and other Internet communication services such as online patient medical records for physicians, but it also has a patient site that includes a medical library and "learning centers" on specific diseases and conditions. Articles come from medical societies and government agencies and are ranked as general-, advanced-, or professional-level resources. The site also contains medical illustrations and a collection of Spanish-language articles.

PatientINFORM
www.patientinform.org
PatientINFORM is a new collaboration between some scientific research journals and voluntary organizations like the American Cancer Society. The journals offer access to new research papers about a disease or condition through the organization's Web site, while the organization itself provides an easy-to-read explanation of what the new research means and how it might affect your treatment or diagnosis. As of this writing, the American Cancer Society, the American Diabetes Association, and the American Heart Association are the only participating organizations.

American Society of Clinical Oncology (ASCO)
http://www.asco.org
ASCO maintains an extensive Web site that provides up-to-date information about cancer and cancer treatment for patients. For each type of cancer listed on the home page, you can find the latest scientific articles, educational material for the public, as well as information and resources specifically for people living with that disease.

Centers for Disease Control and Prevention
www.cdc.gov/az.do
The Centers for Disease Control and Prevention (CDC), a sister federal agency to the National Institutes of Health and another federal government agency. The CDC site tends to have more scientific and less patient-oriented materials

available, but does contain useful information about broader topics like environmental health, workplace injuries, and international health concerns. The site's A to Z index page is a good place to start your search.

The Stanford Health Library
www.med.stanford.edu/healthlibrary/index.html
The Stanford University Health Library Web site is an excellent source of information for specific conditions, medications, online health videos, e-books on health topics, and general health information translated into dozens of languages.

Other Library Services. Your local hospital may have a medical library and medical librarians on staff to help you with specific information searches. Although you may have to pay fees for photocopying or interlibrary loan, the service can save you time and stress over finding the latest articles about your condition.

Several voluntary organizations offer library services over the phone or Internet. Searches are generally free, but there may be fees for photocopying or mailing. Check out the Alzheimer's Association online library (www.alz.org/Services/LibraryServices .asp) for a good example of this service, as well as appendix G for more information.

I need to find information about treatments.

Sometimes you can read everything you ever wanted to know about the biology of your particular disease and still not understand exactly what is involved in the drugs that your doctor has recommended. Or, you may want more information on two different types of surgery that seem to be the most common treatments for your condition. There are a few resources that can help specifically with procedures and treatments. You can also look at appendix G to see which of the major disease organizations offer decision support tools and treatment guides.

One way to get acquainted with the tools available to help you make sense of a treatments' benefits and risks is to use a blank decision form to work through a choice you are facing. It will ask you to describe the options, identify the pros and cons of each, and assign values to them. A blank form can be found in an interactive Web-based format, or as a PDF file, at the Ottawa Health Research Institute's Web site at http://decisionaid.ohri.ca/decguide.html.

The most complete listing of good quality decision aids that are specific to questions about disease treatment and prevention can be found at http://decisionaid.ohri.ca/AZinvent.php.

See the next section for decision tools tied to specific treatments.

Remember: decision aids prepare you to have a discussion with your physician but do not substitute for doing so.

I need more information on how to evaluate
specific procedures and treatments.

Healthfinder
www.healthfinder.gov/
This site, sponsored by the United States Department of Health and Human Services, offers many of the same features as the NIH Health page and MedlinePlus, but does include a useful illustrated guide to diagnostic and surgical procedures. The guide does a good job explaining why a particular procedure is needed ("A biopsy is usually performed to determine if the cells from a sample of body tissue are abnormal.") and answering other simple but important questions such as "How long will it take?" and "Will it hurt?"

MedicineNet.com
www.medicinenet.com
MedicineNet is a general health information site with articles reviewed by a team of doctors. Along with information on specific diseases, the site also contains short descriptions of common medical procedures. The site is owned by the publishers of the *Webster's New World Medical Dictionary*.

Mayo Clinic
www.mayoclinic.com/
The Mayo Clinic's public health site allows you to search for information by disease or condition, with an emphasis on

how to manage your disease. The site also contains decision-making guidance that can help you decide what kind of treatment is best for your condition. Videos and slide shows explain several diseases and medical procedures.

Best Treatments
www.besttreatments.org
The Best Treatments site, which uses information from the *British Medical Journal*, has information on understanding risk, the latest evidence about treatments for a number of conditions, and treatment decision tools you can use with your doctor. Unfortunately, this useful source of information is available only to some patients through their health insurance plans. United HealthCare is one of the bigger plans to subscribe to the service, but check with your plan to see if the site is available to you.

Subimo
www.subimo.com
Subimo is a company that provides online tools for making health-care decisions, from choosing the right prescription medication or insurance plan to finding highly qualified doctors and hospitals that specialize in your condition. Some employers and health-care plans purchase access to the tools for their employees or subscribers, but individuals can also subscribe to the health-care information online tool at a cost of $12 for six months.

Aetna Clinical Policy Bulletin
www.aetna.com/about/cov_det_policies.html
The insurance company Aetna publishes Clinical Policy Bulletins that summarize recent evidence-based research on medications, medical treatments, and even dental treatments, to help physicians decide on a course of action for their patients. The summaries are quite short and usually focus on very specific conditions. The summaries are available free.

National Cancer Institute
Physician Data Query (PDQ)
www.cancer.gov/cancertopics/pdq/cancerdatabase
1 (800) 4-CANCER
Similar to the Aetna bulletins, these short summaries from

NCI review treatment, screening, and prevention, genetic and alternative and complementary medicine research from more than seventy peer-reviewed journals. The summaries are updated monthly and many are available in Spanish. They are freely available at the NCI Web site or by calling the NCI helpline.

I'm still having trouble understanding the technical language of what I'm reading.

If you are intent on collecting all possible information on your diagnosis, you will start running into increasingly complicated jargon and statistics that describe your condition and treatments. The resources below can help you make sense of the gobble-dygook and the suspicious math equations:

American Association for Clinical Chemistry
http://labtestsonline.org/
This site provides a comprehensive list of laboratory tests and the terminology used for each.

Short Course in Medical Terminology
www.dmu.edu/medterms/
The Des Moines University site walks users through medical terms related to specific diseases, and contains quizzes to test your knowledge about what you've just learned.

Medical Dictionary for Kids
Nemours Foundation
www.kidshealth.org/kid/word/index.html
This medical glossary was written specifically for children. For instance, "acne" is described as "little red bumps on the skin called pimples." The site would be useful for children with a serious diagnosis or for explaining an adult's diagnosis to a child (see chapter 3).

How do risk numbers relate to me and my condition?

When you read in a newspaper article that a new cancer drug increases the risk of serious side effects by 45 percent, what does

that number really mean? These Web pages can help you understand the basic statistics of medical risk. It is helpful to read several of these pages, since each page explains the concepts in a
slightly different way.

National Institute on Aging
www.niapublications.org/tipsheets/risk.asp
This short article on risk explains what health researchers
mean by absolute and relative risk and describes the different types of medical studies used to come up with these
numbers.

Breastcancer.org
Weighing Pros and Cons of Treatments
www.breastcancer.org/treatment_stats.html
This page from the nonprofit breastcancer.org site describes
relative and absolute risk in terms of how to decide which
breast cancer treatment might be best suited for you.

Aetna's Intelihealth
www.intelihealth.com/IH/ihtIH/WSIHW000/35320/35323/327
387.html?d=dmtHMSContent
This short article describes relative and absolute risks, but
also discusses the difference between small, early studies of a
treatment and larger-scale studies carried out over several
years. The article also talks about why certain factors can be
associated with a disease but are not the cause of a disease.

GeneticHealth.com
www.genetichealth.com/Risk_Tutorial.shtml
This Web page discusses risk and chance with the help of
numerous pictures, including the types of graphs that you
might come across in a medical study.

*I'm still not sure if the information I'm collecting
is really reliable and accurate.*

The Internet can be a gold mine for health information seekers,
but separating the accurate and useful sites from sites run by
people trying to sell you something, sites created by people
who aren't qualified to give technical information, and sites that

contain outright fraud and misinformation, make the online world more of a land mine in some cases. The following sites can help you determine whether what you're reading is unbiased and based on scientific evidence.

MedlinePlus's guide to "healthy" Websurfing is at www.nlm .nih.gov/medlineplus/healthywebsurfing.html. In addition, try:

Ix for Consumers
www.ixcenter.org/consumers/
The Information Therapy for Consumers Web site offers general advice about finding evidence-based medical information, including counseling services and clinical trials, on the Internet.

Medical Library Association
www.mlanet.org/resources/userguide.html
The MLA site contains information on how to evaluate health Web sites and recommendations for the top 10 Web sites for cancer, diabetes, and heart disease information.

National Human Genome Research Institute
www.genome.gov/11008303#2
This NIH site, designed to help people with rare genetic disorders, briefly discusses the different types of scientific studies and what kind of information they are best at providing. The site has links to some of the other NIH Web pages on evaluating health information, and it also contains links to sites that explain how Internet search engines work.

National Cancer Institute
www.cancer.gov/cancertopics/factsheet/Information/internet
NCI's fact sheet about evaluating health information on the Internet gives tips for determining whether a Web site is potentially biased, unreliable, or out-of-date, and explains how the Food and Drug Administration and the Federal Trade Commission are trying to cut down on fraud on health Web sites.

Health Compass
www.healthcompass.org
This site from the American Federation for Aging Research and the Merck Institute of Aging and Health is designed

especially to help older people navigate the Internet in search of health information. The site provides information on Internet searching, evaluating Web pages, and planning a course of action after researching your condition.

Sense about Science
www.senseaboutscience.org.uk/peerreview/
"I Don't Know What to Believe..." is a short pamphlet published by a British nonprofit organization promoting public understanding of science. The pamphlet explains scientific peer review and how to recognize a good scientific journal article.

> *I heard on the news about a new treatment and*
> *I want to find out how credible it is.*

www.HealthNewsReview.org
This Web site is a program of the Foundation for Informed Decision-making and is published by the University of Minnesota. It grades breaking media reports on new medical findings for accuracy, balance, and completeness.

http://mediadoctor.org.au/
This site is sponsored by the University of Newcastle in Australia. It provides ratings of recent treatment studies, and identifies their strengths and weaknesses.

www.nelh.nhs.uk/hth/archive.asp
This site is sponsored by the National Health Service in the United Kingdom. It critically discussed media coverage of new medical studies.

Top-Ranked Health Web Sites

Forbes and *Consumer Reports* magazines have both created "Best of the Web" lists for top health Web pages, based on the accuracy, usefulness, and timeliness of the Web pages' content.

Forbes Best of the Web
www.forbes.com/bow/b2c/section.jhtml?id=9

Consumer Reports
www.healthratings.org

The Health on the Net Foundation has created a code of conduct (HONcode) that spells out rules for maintaining reliable and credible health information Web sites. Sites that abide by these rules can put the HONcode "seal of approval" on their sites. For more information about the HONcode, go to www.hon.ch/HONcode/.

Books on Family and Illness

For Children and Teens

Can I Still Kiss You? Answering Children's Questions about Cancer by Neil Russell. Deerfield Beach, Florida: HCI Publishers, 2001.

The Grieving Teen: A Guide for Teenagers and Their Friends by Helen Fitzgerald. New York: Fireside, 2001.

Our Family Has Cancer, Too! by Christine Clifford. Minneapolis: University of Minnesota Press, 2002.

What's Wrong with Grandma? A Family's Experience with Alzheimer's by Margaret Shawver. Amherst, New York: Prometheus Books, 1996.

When Mommy Is Sick by Ferne Sherkin-Langer. Morton Grove, Illinois: Albert Whitman & Company, 1995.

For the Whole Family

Alzheimer's Disease: The Family Journey by Wayne A. Caron, James J. Pattee, and Orlo J. Otteson. Plymouth, Minnesota: North Ridge Press, 2001.

American College of Physicians Home Care Guide for HIV and AIDS: For Family and Friends Giving Care at Home, Peter S. Houts, ed. Philadelphia: American College of Physicians 1998.

Cancer in the Family: Helping Children Cope with a Parent's Illness by Sue P. Heiney, Joan F. Hermann, Katherine V. Bruss, and Joy L. Fincannon. Atlanta: American Cancer Society, 2001.

The Etiquette of Illness: What to Say When You Can't Find the Words by Susan Halpern. New York: Bloomsbury, 2004.

Facing Cancer: A Complete Guide for People with Cancer, Their Families, and Caregivers by Theodore A. Stern and Mikkael A. Sekeres. New York: McGraw-Hill Professional, 2003.

How to Help Children Through a Parent's Serious Illness by Kathleen McCue and Ron Bonn. New York: St. Martin's Press, 1994.

Living with Stroke : A Guide For Families: Help and New Hope for All Those Touched by Stroke by Richard C. Senelick, Peter W. Rossi, and Karla Dougherty. Chicago: Contemporary Books, 1999.

Raising an Emotionally Healthy Child When a Parent Is Sick by Paula Rauch and A. C. Muriel. New York: McGraw–Hill, 2006.

Stroke and the Family: A New Guide by Joel Stein. Boston: Harvard University Press, 2004.

Find the Right Doctors and Hospitals

How Do I Start My Doctor Search?

FOR MOST SERIOUS MEDICAL DIAGNOSES, you will need to see a specialist for your condition. If you have been diagnosed with breast cancer and need to have a tumor surgically removed, for instance, you should choose a doctor with specific expertise in breast surgery. In many cases, getting a referral from your primary care doctor will be the first step toward finding the right kind of specialist.

Your local hospital will almost certainly have a referral service that you can call to get names of local physicians who treat your condition. Just be aware that most hospital referral services only give out the names of doctors that have privileges at the hospital. You could also search in the phone book or online for local physicians' societies that offer physician finder services. (Check the San Francisco Medical Society (www.sfms .org/) or the Wyoming Medical Society (www.wyomed.org) for examples.)

Books with updated lists of physicians around the country are usually available at your local library or bookstore. In most cases, the information in the books is pretty brief—just a listing of the doctor's name, education, and current specialty. Some of the bigger titles include:

America's Top Doctors: Choosing the Best in Healthcare, 4th edition. Castle Connolly, 2004.
Directory of Physicians in the United States. American Medical Association, 2005. *The Official ABMS Directory of Board Certified Medical Specialists.* American Board of Medical Specialties, 2005.

You can also search for doctors at a variety of Web sites. Some good places to start include:

The American Medical Association
www.ama-assn.org
Click on "DoctorFinder."

The National Library of Medicine Directories Page
www.nlm.nih.gov/medlineplus/directories.html
A great resource for finding a specialist through his or her
professional society.

Medicare.gov
www.medicare.gov/
Click on "Find a Doctor" under "Search Tools."

The National Institute on Aging
www.niapublications.org/engagepages/choose.asp
This organization also has a site on choosing a doctor, with
a thorough list of questions and links to medical associations that can provide more information on particular
specialties.

Medicare
www.medicare.gov
The Medicare site has a pamphlet on choosing a doctor for
Medicare patients at www.medicare.gov/Publications/Pubs/
pdf/10180.pdf. The pamphlet is also available by calling 1
(800) MEDICARE.

WebMD
www.webmd.com/
Click on "Find a Doctor."

For a slightly different take on how to choose a doctor, check
"Finding Mr. Right" by Judy Foreman (*Boston Globe Magazine*, De-
cember 5, 2004) and "To Find a Good Doctor, Ask a Nurse: More
Advice from Medical Insiders" by Tara Parker Pope (*The Wall Street
Journal*, February 10, 2004).

Choosing a Doctor

There are a few basic questions that everyone should ask before
choosing a doctor, no matter how much or how little you want to
research your physician:

- Does the doctor have the right expertise? See "How Do I Start My Doctor Search," page 206. Physicians who are specially trained to treat your condition can make a difference in your care.

- Does the doctor participate in your insurance plan? Unfortunately, most people don't have the resources that allow them to pick any doctor out of the thousands that are available. If you have health insurance, your insurance provider probably has a list of physicians whose work is covered under your plan. This doesn't necessarily mean that you are restricted to only those physicians, but check your personal plan to find out how much you might have to pay out of pocket if you do use a doctor off the "preferred" list.

- At what hospital does your doctor have privileges? A doctor's privileges at a hospital simply means that the doctor is allowed to practice at that hospital. If you have a serious diagnosis, you may need to visit a specific hospital in your city or county to get treatment. If at all possible, you want your doctor to be available to treat you at that hospital.

- What does the grapevine say? It doesn't hurt to listen to what your friends, family, neighbors, hairdresser, or mechanic might know about a particular doctor, as long as you take such advice with a grain of salt. Remember that your diagnosis is unique—a surgeon who "worked miracles" on your cousin might not be able to do the same for you, simply because your condition will be different from his. Your personality and approach to your illness is also unique—everyone you speak to may warn you away from a "heartless" oncologist, but you might find her manner to be straightforward and businesslike, just what you were hoping for.

- All else being equal, I don't want to ride the bus. If all else truly seems equal (though it rarely is), you may want to choose a doctor who is convenient to your home or work or who has the best office hours for you. As you're already finding out, managing your illness is stressful enough. You

> may not want to add an hour's drive through rush hour
> traffic or a commit to regular long trips to the nearest city
> in iffy winter weather into the mix.

After you've answered these basic questions, choose one of the approaches below to learn a little or a lot more about a potential doctor.

The Minimal Approach: I'm Happy with My Referral, but I Just Want to Check a Few Things...

EDUCATION

Using one of the physician finder resources mentioned above, double-check your doctor's education. All medical schools in the United States that grant medical degrees and degrees in osteo-pathic medicine (a whole-body approach to medicine that stresses the interconnectedness of the body's systems) are accredited by a group called the Liaison Committee for Medical Education, and are usually accredited by state agencies and other accreditation groups for colleges and universities.

The standards for medical schools outside the United States vary, but all foreign medical graduates must pass the same exams that students in the United States take to become licensed physicians.

BOARD CERTIFICATION

Doctors are "board certified" when they have completed a training program and exam testing their knowledge in a particular specialty. The American Board of Medical Specialties (ABMS) can tell you whether your doctor is board certified in any of twenty-four specialties, from allergies to urology. You can get this information from ABMS's Web site at www.abms.org (Click on "Who's Certi-fied," and complete the free e-mail registration); or through their certification phone hotline at (866) ASK–ABMS, or in *The Official ABMS Directory of Board Certified Medical Specialists*.

The ABMS also has a helpful FAQ at its Web site that answers questions such as "What does it mean to be 'board eligible?'" and "Are chiropractors board certified?" The FAQ can be found at www.abms.org/faq.asp.

You can also find board certification information through many doctor finder services, such as the American Medical Association's Web site (see page 207).

DISCIPLINARY ACTION

Doctors can be disciplined by their state medical licensing boards for problems ranging from a failure to keep up with their continuing education requirements to substance abuse and sexual misconduct. "Discipline" can mean a fine or a reprimand, or, in the most serious cases, suspension or revocation of a doctor's license to practice medicine. Disciplinary action does *not* include malpractice claims (see below). There are several sources you can consult to find out if your doctor has been disciplined by a state medical licensing board.

> Federation of State Medical Boards
> www.docinfo.org
> The Federation of State Medical Boards
> Attn: Physician Profiles
> PO Box 972507
> Dallas, Texas 75397-2507

For $9.95, you can use the FSMB's Web site or mail in a request to find out if there have been any disciplinary actions taken against a doctor.

You can also contact your state's medical board directly to find out about a doctor's disciplinary status. Be aware, however, that some medical boards will not release any information about pending disciplinary charges against a physician. To find a list of phone numbers and Web sites for state boards, go to the American Medical Association Web site: www.ama-assn.org and type "state medical boards" into the search box to find contact information for your state.

MALPRACTICE

Information on a doctor's malpractice suits and judgments are often difficult to dig up, particularly if legal action is ongoing. Some state medical boards collect information on malpractice, but it is not always available to the public. If your local library has free access to LexisNexis, a premier online legal database, you may be able to search for court cases by your doctor's name. Some of the more intensive doctor search services listed below will also research malpractice judgments for you.

A few things to remember about medical malpractice:

- Some specialties such as obstetrics, emergency medicine, and surgery are more prone to malpractice suits, so comparing the number of malpractice suits brought against a surgeon compared to a family doctor is not always very helpful in choosing a doctor.

- Don't assume that a doctor' payment in a malpractice suit is an admission of guilt. Some doctors prefer to settle suits to avoid other costly legal bills or to try to keep their malpractice insurance rates within a certain level.

- Details and trends are important. If you can get access to a doctor's malpractice suit records, try to find out whether the suits repeatedly refer to one specific procedure, or if the records point out a pattern of negligence rather than isolated mistakes.

The Maximum Approach: The More Information, the Better

Some people want to know as much as possible about the doctors they choose for their care, including any available information about how they rank compared to other area doctors in quality care, whether they have been involved in any malpractice actions, how long they have practiced in a particular specialty, and other details. If you want to dig deeper before settling on a doctor, there are several sources for those extra details. The information in these more extensive doctor profiles may not be free and may require you to provide information about yourself that you would prefer to keep private, including your address or details about your condition.

National Committee for Quality Assurance (NCQA)
www.ncqa.org/PhysicianQualityReports.htm
The NCQA is a nonprofit organization that collects

information on the quality of managed health-care programs
in the United States. For NCQA, "quality" means how well
physicians meet certain standards of care for particular diseases or conditions, such as whether they use the best and
most recent medical evidence in their treatment decisions.
The Web site allows you to search by state to find doctors in
your area that have been recognized as quality caregivers for
particular conditions like stroke and diabetes.

HealthGrades
www.healthgrades.com/
1 (303) 716-0041
HealthGrades is a for-profit health-care quality ratings company, offering reports on more than 600,000 individual doctors. The doctor report cards list education, specialty, board
certification, any disciplinary actions taken by the state in
the past five years, the doctor's gender, and any foreign languages she or he speaks, and compares the doctor's education, years in practice, and disciplinary record to other
physicians in the same specialty and all physicians nationwide. The report also contains a brief section on quality
rankings of nearby hospitals and general questions to ask
before choosing a doctor. Much of the information contained in each report can be found free elsewhere, but the
service conveniently collects it all into one report, making it
easy to compare doctors. Physician reports cost $7.95, and
$2.95 for each additional report in one order.

ChoiceTrust
www.choicetrust.com
ChoiceTrust is another for-profit consumer directory that
provides reports on physicians nationwide, using information from publicly available databases and compiling them
in one place. The service provides essentially the same information as HealthGrades, but without the hospital quality
data or physician comparisons. However, it might be a good
place to look if you can't find a particular doctor on Health-
Grades. Searching for a physician is free, individual physician reports cost $7.95, and a 24-hour day pass for the site
with unlimited access to reports is $11.95.

Consumers' CHECKBOOK Guide to Top Doctors
www.checkbook.org/doctors/pageone.cfm
1 (800) 213-7283
Consumers' CHECKBOOK, a nonprofit consumer organization based in Washington, D.C., publishes a listing of 20,000 "top doctors" nationally, based on what specialist doctors themselves say they would recommend for their loved ones. Along with information about board certification, location, and specialty, the guide also tallies how many times each doctor was recommended by others. The book (or online access to the database for two years) costs $24.95.

Best Doctors
www.bestdoctors.com
1 (800) 223-5003
Best Doctors, a for-profit group, has compiled a list of 50,000 top doctors around the country as the basis of a consultation service that it offers to employers and health insurance carriers. If your employer or insurer subscribes to their program, its clinicians can review your medical records, confirm diagnoses, and recommend specific treatments to your own doctor.

Doctor Evidence
www.doctorevidence.com
1 (888) 633-2822
As part of its evidence-based research service (see appendix A), Doctor Evidence offers "concierge service"—a customized search for the best specialists, treatment, and diagnostic centers for your specific condition. Cost of the service varies depending on the nature of your condition and the hours spent in research by the company.

Castle Connolly Medical Research Inc.
Doctor-Patient Advisor
www.castleconnolly.com/advisory.cfm
1 (212) 367-8400 x16
Castle Connolly, the publishers of *America's Top Doctors*, also offers Doctor-Patient Advisor, a one-on-one consultation service that pairs patients with a physician or specialty-trained nurse who helps them find an appropriate specialist. The service costs $275.

Among the most expensive ways to find a doctor are "personal patient advocate services," which for a substantial fee will research the top specialists for you, handle your appointment, test, and insurance paperwork, and even help you bypass a doctor's waiting list.

Planning for Surgery

If you are facing surgery, you may want to do some background work before you commit fully, first, because surgical techniques vary depending on the surgeon and institution, and you may have more choices than you realize; second, because the experience of the hospital and the surgeon and the surgical team can influence the outcome of the surgery; third, because the cost of surgery varies across institutions; and fourth, because surgery is a big deal and it is helpful to know what to expect.

The book *Second Opinion: The Columbia Presbyterian Guide to Surgery* by Eric Rose (New York: St. Martin's Press, 2000) provides a comprehensive approach to evaluating your surgical options as well as finding the right surgeon for your needs.

A number of Web sites provide information about different aspects of surgery you may want to consider:

Agency for Healthcare Research and Quality
http://ahrq.gov/consumer/index.html
AHRQ is the federal agency whose mandate includes improving the quality and safety of health care. The surgery sections guidance about planning and what you need to know about surgery.

American College of Surgeons
www.facs.org/public_info/patentinfo.html
This Web site answers frequently asked questions, offers information about common operations and provides guidance about choice of surgeon, cost of surgery, and how to talk about fees with your doctor.

American College of Anesthesiologists
www.asahq.org/patienteducation.htm
The Web site of this professional association provides valuable information about anesthesia and sedation and

discusses which types are used for what purposes as well as postsurgical pain control.

Choosing a Hospital

Hospital rankings and ratings have become more widely available in the last five years, thanks to the efforts of evidence-based medicine supporters such as the NCQA and the Leapfrog Group, a group of companies and other health-care insurance purchasers who have agreed to buy health care that meets certain safety and quality standards. Although you might not be able to freely choose a hospital if your specialist has privileges in only one place, your insurance only applies to certain facilities, or if you can't travel far, it can be helpful to know whether there are any differences in the possibilities available to you.

The Leapfrog Group
www.leapfroggroup.org
1 (202) 292-6713
The Leapfrog Group's quality and safety ratings are available free online. The ratings measure hospitals' performance in areas such as patient safety, technology, high risk proce-dures, and intensive care, rather than specific procedures or diseases. Leapfrog uses information that hospitals report vol-untarily, so the ratings may not be available for all hospitals in your area.

Quality Check—Joint Commission on Accreditation of Healthcare Organizations
www.jcaho.org/quality+check/index.htm
JCAHO is the nation's leading nonprofit accreditation group that encourages quality and safety standards among health-care facilities and gives a seal of approval to those that meet its standards. Quality Check is JCAHO's online search service of accredited hospitals, laboratories, nursing homes, and even outpatient care such as sleep clinics.

HealthGrades
www.healthgrades.com/
1 (303) 716-0041
Along with its physician report cards, HealthGrades produces

report cards for more than five thousand facilities. Health-Grades offers free information on how well hospitals in your area rate on twenty-eight common medical conditions or procedures. More detailed reports on individual hospitals, including safety ratings, the average length of stay in the hospital, and cost of common procedures, are available for $9.95, and $2.95 for each additional report in one order.

Hospital Compare
www.hospitalcompare.hhs.gov/
This government Web site allows you to search for Medicare-certified hospitals in your area and find out about how well they rate in terms of quality care for heart attack, heart failure, and pneumonia, compared to other hospitals nationwide. The site is easy to navigate, but detailed information on individual hospitals is sparse.

Performance Ratings for Hospitals in California—California HealthCare Foundation
www.calhospitals.org
This Web site rates California hospitals based on patients' perceptions of their treatment, including emotional support by staff, physical comfort, respect for patient preference, and how well the staff involved family and friends. The site also contains an excellent, step-by-step guide to choosing a hospital.

U.S. News & World Report—Best Hospitals 2005
www.usnews.com/usnews/health/best-hospitals/tophosp.htm
U.S. News & World Report ranks hospitals nationwide according to the hospitals' performance in seventeen specialty fields, from cancer to psychiatry. The rankings are based on reputation (from a survey of board-certified doctors in a particular specialty), death rates, and other factors such as the number of nurses assigned to each patient and the use of important technologies for a particular specialty.

PATIENT SAFETY
The news is full of reports on problems with patient safety and medical errors occurring in the hospital. This has sparked a re-

sponse from the government to help patients protect themselves. The Agency for Healthcare Research and Quality has a number of pamphlets and tip sheets available on topics that will help people prepare for encounters with acute care. See www.ahrq.gov/ CONSUMER/ and scroll down to the section titled "Quality."

Clinical Trials and Second Opinion Services

Clinical Trials

CLINICAL TRIALS ARE RESEARCH STUDIES with people—instead of mice or cells in a test tube—as the focus of the study. Clinical trials can test a new drug, a new surgical technique, or even a new type of alternative therapy, such as meditation, to determine whether the treatment is safe and effective. By definition, the treatment is untested, so there may be some risk to participating in a trial. However, patients can often get access to promising treatments in their early stages by enrolling in clinical trials.

A good place to start learning about clinical trials is the National Institutes of Health Web site ClinicalTrials.gov. (www.clinicaltrials .gov) This comprehensive site includes a short discussion of what clinical trials are and how they work, including the benefits and risks of participating in a trial, the process of informed consent (see chapter 6), and how patients are chosen for specific trials.

In addition, the Web site allows users to search for both recently completed and ongoing government funded and privately funded clinical trials in which you may be able to participate. You can search the trials database on the site by keywords such as "heart attack," the name of your condition, the organization or company sponsoring the trial, and the geographical location of the trial.

The information is only available on the Web, but you can request assistance in using the database from the National Library of Medicine at 1 (888) FINDNLM.

Other government agencies such as the National Cancer Institute maintain their own Web pages for clinical trial searches. In most cases, their databases overlap with the information found in ClinicalTrials.gov, but in some cases information about new trials may be posted more quickly on individual agency sites.

National Cancer Institute
www.cancer.gov/clinical_trials/

Department of Health and Human Services—HIV/AIDS page
http://aidsinfo.nih.gov/clinical_trials/

National Heart, Lung and Blood Institute
www.nhlbi.nih.gov/studies/index.htm

National Institute of Neurological Disorders and Stroke
www.ninds.nih.gov/disorders/clinicaltrials_us.htm

The American Cancer Society (ACS)
www.cancer.org/docroot/ETO/content/ETO_6_3_Clinical_
Trials_-_Patient_Participation.asp
ACS offers a lengthy but easy to read explanation of clinical
trials and what you should consider before participating in
one.

WebMD
http://my.webmd.com/content/pages/13/65814.htm?z=1104_0
8950_8900_ct_01
The WebMD site also has a good discussion of clinical trials
that overlaps somewhat with the ACS site.

Second Opinion Services

Before the Internet, second opinion services were confined mostly
to hospitals, but they are still the most popular option for most
patients seeking additional opinions after recommendations from
their physician and friends and family. Hospital-based second
opinion services generally offer to send your health record and
diagnosis for review to members of their staff who specialize in
your condition.

The plus sides of hospital-based services are that they are
local, they are often free unless you schedule a face-to-face appointment with one of the hospital's specialists and they are relatively easy to use. In most cases, you can arrange for a review of
your records with one short phone call.

On the minus side, the services rarely send your records to
doctors who do not have privileges with the hospital. If your condition is rare, or if specialists for your condition are rare in your

area, the hospital-based service may not be able to track down a useful second opinion. Second opinions offered through the service may lack a lot of details, since they are based only on your records and not on an actual exam.

Internet second opinion services have multiplied rapidly in the past five years. These services usually offer a second opinion on your diagnosis within a specified number of days after they receive a copy of your medical record and items such as your pathology slides from a cancer biopsy. Depending on the service, your records could be reviewed by specialists at a specific hospital, physicians around the country or around the world who specialize in your condition, or a full team of doctors recruited especially for the Internet service. In some cases, the service may also schedule follow-up appointments or further tests with the reviewing doctors with other specialists in your area of the country. You can find a few examples of Internet-based second opinion services below:

Partners Online Specialty Consultations
http://econsults.partners.org
This service from Partners Healthcare in Massachusetts provides a second opinion to your doctor within a week after receiving your record and test results from you and your physician. Prices for the consulations range from $225 to $750, depending on whether a specialist reviews your record.

The Cleveland Clinic
www.clevelandclinic.org/services/eclinic.htm
The Cleveland Clinic, a longtime provider of specialist care and second opinions, has a second opinion service through its e-Cleveland Clinic site. A second opinion, delivered electronically, costs $565.

Find Cancer Experts
http://findcancerexperts.com/
This site offers free reviews of your pathology report by a nationwide network of pathologists. There is a fee (usually $200–$300) for professional review of your actual pathology slides.

A Short Course on Medical Privacy

PROTECTING PRIVACY IN HEALTH CARE is important. You must have some degree of control about who sees your health information so that you can confide in your doctors and so that you can provide them with all of the information they need to make good decisions about your care. If you are selective about the information you provide to your doctor and do not tell her facts that make you vulnerable, you undermine your chances of getting the best care.

You have the right to make decisions about who knows and who doesn't know about your condition. You may want the support that comes with telling friends and colleagues about your condition. Or you may want to present yourself as someone who doesn't have MS or AIDS. This is your choice.

Part of making it your choice is exercising these options about privacy. To begin with, you need to know what your basic privacy rights are under HIPAA.

In general, you must be notified in writing about a doctor's or clinic's policy on sharing health information. You have the right to obtain your health record and ask to have corrections made to your record. Under the rule, a hospital or doctor has to get your written consent to hand over any of your information to your employer or a third party such as an advertising group. You can ask to get sensitive information delivered to you in a way that you choose, such as a phone call instead of mail. You can find out who has accessed your medical record each year. Perhaps most important, you can file a complaint if you think any of these rights have been violated.

The single most consumer-friendly resource about the privacy of medical information can be found at The Privacy Project, www.healthprivacy.org or by calling 1 (202) 721-5632. In addition to basic facts about HIPPA, there is information about your rights at federal and state levels, how to protect your privacy, useful checklists and easy-to-follow guidance about how to file a complaint, should you need to do so.

You can find a complete text of the HIPAA rule at the Department of Health and Human Services Web site at www.hhs .gov/ocr/hipaa/ or by calling the Office of Civil Rights toll-free hotline at 1 (800) 368-1019.

The extensive Web page includes fact sheets on your rights guaranteed under HIPAA, the full text of the HIPAA rule and how the privacy rules apply to research clinical trials and alcohol and drug abuse programs. The site also explains how to file a complaint with the Office of Civil Rights and provides complaint forms if you think your privacy rights under HIPAA have been violated.

If you've read all the information on the official government site and still have questions about exactly what kinds of information are protected and who exactly still has access to your information, the following Web sites are a good source of answers and places to call with questions about your specific situation.

Privacy Rights Clearinghouse
www.privacyrights.org/fs/fs8a-hipaa.htm
1 (619) 298-3396
The nonprofit consumer organization Privacy Rights Clearinghouse has compiled an extensive list of "frequently asked questions" about HIPAA, what the legal language means in plain English and how to protect your medical information.

Electronic Privacy Information Center
www.epic.org/privacy/medical/#federalLaw
EPIC has a Web page with an overview of federal and state laws regarding medical privacy, including information on genetic data privacy and regular updates on medical privacy issues in the news.

American Civil Liberties Union
www.aclu.org/Privacy/Privacy.cfm?ID=13143&c=27
The ACLU Web site contains two pages on how much access your family and friends may have to your medical records under HIPAA, and how much access the federal government has to your medical records under HIPAA and the U.S. Patriot Act.

Medical Information Bureau
www.mib.com/html/consumer.html
1 (866) 692–6901
If you have applied for individually underwritten life, health, or disability insurance within the past seven years, you may have a record with the Medical Insurance Bureau. The MIB compiles individual health data that people provide to insurance companies when seeking coverage. The MIB keeps individual records for seven years. You can get a copy of your MIB record for free once a year by calling the toll-free number above, and can work with MIB to correct any item on your personal report that you feel is in error.

A Guide to Health Professionals

THE SPECIALIST PHYSICIANS who will coordinate your care are directing their efforts toward stopping the progression of your disease and managing its impact on your body. But your diagnosis has reverberated through all aspects of your life—your relationships with family members, your management of daily routines and your emotional equilibrium. Should you feel stuck or at a loss about how to proceed, there are professionals who can help you accommodate to these changes. Here is an annotated list of such professionals, what they offer, and where you might find them.

If you are in distress but are bewildered about the kind of help you need, you may want to look at the "Distress Treatment Guidelines for Patients," available from the American Cancer Society (www.cancer.org; type "distress" in the search box, or call 1–800–ACS–2345) and the National Comprehensive Cancer Network. This booklet includes self-tests and guidance for decisions about treatment.

Out of the hospital

- Primary care provider
- Advice nurse/health coach
- Disease management staff
- Case manager
- Pastoral counselor
- Mental health professional
- Patient advocate
- Financial planner

In the hospital

- Patient navigator

- Case manager

- Medical social worker

- Nurses

- Clergy/health-care chaplain

- Consultation-liaison psychiatrist

- Patient advocate

Out of Hospital

PRIMARY CARE PROVIDER

A primary care provider is the health professional who is your "usual" doctor, the one who knows you and your family, who you call about your earache or a persistent cough, and who has a cumulative sense of your health history. This person can be a primary care physician, a family doctor, an internist, a nurse practitioner, or a specialist like a gynecologist or urologist who has agreed to help you out with some of your other health concerns.

Having a primary care provider who follows you over time has become less common than it was a decade ago. Nevertheless, when you receive a serious diagnosis, she can be of invaluable help to you, even though you probably feel that the last thing you need right now is another doctor. (Take another look at chapter 2, which includes reasons to be in touch with a primary care provider during this time.)

Things it may be helpful to know about
primary care providers

Patients often expect their primary care provider to automatically know about their diagnosis, as though the world of medicine is completely wired and communicating with itself at all times. It isn't. *A specialist will not notify your primary care provider of your diagnosis,* despite the fact that you wrote her name on your form and you talked to your specialist about your primary care doctor. If you want your primary care provider to know about your situation, *you* must tell him or her.

If you want to have a real conversation about your condition with your provider, make an appointment to see him rather than doing so on the telephone. Unless you are a member of a staff model HMO, it is likely that your primary care provider works alone or in a group practice and is thus a small business person working on a slim margin. For the most part, health insurance doesn't cover telephone conversations but does cover office visits. You want your provider's undivided attention.

Nurse practitioners are primary care providers who are trained to take a holistic approach to their patients, i.e., to address their medical needs while being particularly aware of how illness affects their abilities to manage everyday tasks. So, for example, a nurse practitioner will be attuned to symptom management and nutritional aspects of different conditions, as well as the impact of medication side effects on a patient's ability to walk or work or drive. Nurse practitioners also focus on the transitions in the lives of their patients. "Nursing is about facilitating transitions from one stable period to another," said Afaf Meleis, Dean of Nursing at the University of Pennsylvania. "Nurse practitioners are well connected in their communities and can identify the services and professionals a family needs to accommodate to a new serious diagnosis."

ADVICE NURSE / HEALTH COACH

Many hospitals, health plans, and some employers have purchased telephone services that allow members and employees to call a telephone number to speak to a nurse. The idea behind these phone lines is the notion that you can take action to improve your health or care for an illness without seeing a doctor, if you have access to experts who can provide the critical information to help you make the right decisions.

That said, there are big differences in the training and orientation of the people who answer those telephone health lines.

Many are *advice nurses,* who focus on providing information, answering questions, and giving advice ranging from steps you can take to stop smoking to whether you should take your child to the emergency room for his earache or if it is safe to wait and see the doctor in the morning.

There are other health professionals—mostly nurses—who are trained as health "coaches." The aim of the health coach is to help the caller think through health decisions and to give patients the skills to think about what they need to do—should you seek another opinion for your diagnosis of ALS? Where? What can you expect about the pace of decline in your husband's Parkinson's disease and are there things besides drugs that might slow it down? Who knows this and how do you get to them?

Don't assume your plan has a coaching component—some plans don't differentiate between advice and coaching. But this is a free service and might give you the answers to some of the little questions that are bugging you. Call the number with health questions that arise in the course of your day and see how helpful they are to you.

DISEASE MANAGEMENT PROGRAMS

Some serious highly prevalent conditions may trigger referral to a disease management program that is part of your health-care benefit. Although the people I talked with for this book were rarely referred to disease management programs within the time frame the book covers, you may wish to inquire of your health plan if they have a disease management program for members with your diagnosis.

Such programs may offer good access to oncology nurses, for example, who can be helpful in answering questions and talking with you about information you have tracked down elsewhere about medication and managing symptoms and side effects.

CASE MANAGER

Certain diagnoses and levels of spending will result in your health plan or insurance company assigning a case manager to you. Case managers are usually nurses and their job is to make sure you get evidence-based health care.

On one hand, case managers work for the company and their job is to make sure you get the best care at a reasonable cost and don't receive care that is not deemed "medically necessary."

Sometimes the net effect may be that you feel that you are getting booted out of the hospital while you are still far too ill to be at home or can't get a medicine or service that you need.

On the other hand, as nurses, they are deeply committed to their patients and they can be valuable allies in trying to solve the problem of how to get the best care for your condition. They know everything about your health plan and how to get services covered. They can be an excellent resource in solving day-to-day problems and a valuable ally in advocating for you with your health plan.

If you think you would benefit from a case manager, call your health plan and inquire if you can get one assigned to you.

When your case manager contacts you, approach this news with the idea that you have an additional resource available to you and that together, you can solve the problem of how to get the care you need. The attitude that this person is going to approve only the minimal services and values saving money more than your life is going to start you off on the wrong foot.

To find out if your insurance company's case managers are accredited by an organization that monitors the quality and standards of case management nationwide, you can check their credentials with the nonprofit group URAC, which evaluates the quality of health-care programs. Their online directory of accredited case management programs is available at www.urac.org/prog_directory_main.asp.

PASTORAL COUNSELOR

People who identify with a religious tradition or who are a member of a faith community may find comfort in talking with clergy from their own denomination—often someone they know, and who knows them and their family.

But sometimes that familiarity gets in the way: Some people fear that if they tell their priest or rabbi about their diagnosis that they will get an answer like "I'll pray for you" or "It's in God's hands." If you expect this is what you will hear and don't think it will be helpful, you may not want go to your minister or priest. Similarly, if you are questioning your faith or are struggling to bring your spiritual resources to bear on this crisis, you may be uncomfortable or concerned about asking for scarce attention over time.

Certified pastoral counselors are clergy and lay religious professionals who have been trained as clinical social workers or
counselors or psychotherapists. Some work for congregations but
most work in counseling centers or on their own. Reverend
George Handzo, a HealthCare chaplain with the HealthCare Chap-
laincy in New York City describes the orientation of pastoral
counselors like this: "We believe each person has the resources
within them to confront what is happening to them—our job is
to help them to find those resources.

"People want a relationship with God: We believe that they
want someone who is willing to walk with them in the valley of
the shadow of death. This doesn't mean that God is going to keep
them out of that valley, but they don't want to be alone. And if
we can help them reestablish their relationship with God as
someone who will walk with them through this crisis, then we've
allowed them to find the strength and ability to move on to the
other things they must do. It is not an insult to God and not blas-
phemous to ask the question; 'How could you do this to me?'"

Simkha Weintraub, a rabbi, psychologist, and the director
of the Center for Jewish Healing in New York City, says, "People
know when they get that diagnosis that they are entering a new
identity and they need a new language and fellow travelers.
That's what they call about. They are looking for someone who
understands but who gets the health crisis part."

It is important to note that pastoral counseling is based on allowing each person to have his or her own view of God. As part
of becoming certified, counselors sign a code of ethics that includes a prohibition against proselytizing.

If you do choose to talk with a pastoral counselor, interview
her in the same way you would interview a doctor—ask what
experience she has working with your condition.

The American Association of Pastoral Counselors has a directory of counselors at its Web site (www.aapc.org) or you can ask
for a referral in your area by calling 1 (703) 385-6967. Counseling
services are usually not free.

MENTAL HEALTH PROFESSIONALS
If you feel so overwhelmed and confused that you don't know
what direction to go, are experiencing overwhelming anxiety,

are having difficulty sleeping, are irritable and angry, are barking at family members or panicking, you may want to get a little help.

Sometimes people don't have anyone to talk to about their fears—they don't want to talk with their spouse or kids or partners about it because they don't want to seem ungrateful or to discourage them or show that they are frightened.

An excellent counselor, regardless of his training as a clinical social worker, mental health counselor, psychologist, or psychiatrist, is what you are looking for.

If you already have a relationship with a counselor or psychotherapist, this is a good time to get in touch with him or her. A professional who already knows you knows where you are vulnerable and can provide valuable support during this time.

But beware the mental health professional who is either completely unfamiliar with your disease or who seems upset by it. There are psychiatrists, psychologists, clinical nurse specialists, counselors, and social workers who are trained to understand your reaction to your specific diagnosis. If you are starting your search from the beginning, consider looking for professionals who are trained to work with people who are medically ill.

They understand the urgency of your situation. They won't give you an appointment for six weeks from now. They will want to talk about what is going on with you *now* and how this illness is affecting you, rather than excavating your history and exploring long–term problems. They will know how to help you distinguish the symptoms of the disease from the symptoms of your upset. They will be able to figure out if you are depressed and could benefit from medication. They will be able to identify potential interactions between medicine you are taking for your disease and those you may take for anxiety or depression.

The approach these professionals will take is different from regular psychotherapy. It is more action oriented. It involves developing a rapid positive connection with the therapist around concerns related to your medical situation. The conversation will begin with your medical situation, rather than "tell me about your childhood." It is directed and focused on your crisis.

There are several places to start your search for a mental health professional if you do not get a referral from your other doctors:

American Psychosocial Oncology Society
www.APOS-society.org
1 (866) 276-7443
The society provides local referral for counseling through its hotline message service, which is checked three times a day. The Web site also contains a directory of local professionals (www.apos-society.org/survivors/helpline/provider.aspx) who have offered their services through APOS to provide counseling for distressed cancer patients and their families.

American Psychological Association—APA Find a Psychologist
http://locator.apahelpcenter.org/
1 (800) 964-2000 (toll-free)
You can use the Web site to find listings of local psychologists, or the hotline operator can use your zip code to locate and connect you with the referral service of the state psychological association.

American Psychiatric Association
1 (888) 35-PSYCH (toll-free)
The American Psychiatric Association hotline can connect you with the referral service of your district branch of the APA.

Clinical Social Work Federation
nfscswlo@aol.com
You can send an e-mail to the federation to request a confidential referral to a clinical social worker in your state.

American Mental Health Counselors Association
www.find-a-counselor.net/default.htm
1 (877) 956-6400
The Web site and hotline only offer referrals to counselors who have registered with the association's referral service, so referrals may be limited in your area.

Psychology Today—Therapy Directory
http://therapists.psychologytoday.com/rms/prof_search.php
The *Psychology Today* online directory of therapists is searchable by location and condition, and contains contact information and a small blurb written by each therapist on their specialties and approach.

Disease-specific organizations may also offer counseling services or referrals. Check appendix G for more information.

Other referral sources include your local medical college or academic medical center's consultation liaison psychiatry department and your state health department.

PATIENT ADVOCATES

One of the effects of the increasing complexity of health care and insurance is the growth of an unruly jungle of consultants of every variety, willing to off-load aspects of being a full-fledged patient for a fee. Because they are completely unregulated, it is difficult to pass judgment, forewarn, or recommend any in particular.

Here are some of the consultants and consulting firms that people I talked with mentioned using, with mixed success.

- Retired physicians who will conduct research on your condition and its treatment and provide you with recommendations based on the research.

- Nurses, ex-hospital administrators, and trained advocates who will go over every expense on every bill and negotiate with doctors and hospitals and the insurance company.

- Attorneys and former health plan executives who will advise you on appeals to your health insurance company or health plan for reimbursement for uncovered treatments.

- Specially trained nurses and social workers who will advise you on your rights and responsibilities for receiving Medicare, Medicaid, and Social Security, what the benefits are and how to obtain them (this service can often be found for free from community organizations such as the State Medicaid Office, ADRC [Aging and Disability Resource Centers], the State Health Insurance counselors, [Medicare] Medicare carriers, 1–800 Medicare, or the Social Security resource line).

- Former patients whose experience with their illness highlighted the needs of others for advice and support about how to negotiate various aspects of a serious illness.

Increasingly, these consultants have signed on to work with patient advocacy firms and nonprofit centers to provide all these services. While the nonprofit centers usually focus on helping you decide among treatments or sort out insurance billing free, firms usually change a fee ranging from $80 to $250 an hour, while some larger organizations offer "deluxe" services that can come with hefty membership fees of thousands of dollars a year.

A few for-profit patient advocacy centers and firms are listed below. Also, check out appendix G under "Financial, Insurance, and Legal Aid" for similar nonprofit advocacy groups.

The Center for Patient Partnerships at the University of Wisconsin
www.law.wisc.edu/patientadvocacy/
1 (608) 265-6267
The center offers help in understanding your diagnosis, solving insurance snarls and making sense of medical bills, searching for a second opinion, and determining your eligibility for federal and state benefit programs for people with chronic or life-threatening illnesses. The service is offered nationwide free of charge.

Patient Advocate Foundation
www.patientadvocate.org
1 (800) 532-5274
The Patient Advocate Foundation is a nonprofit organization that can work with insurers, creditors, and employers on coverage appeals, employee benefits, and bill payment. The foundation also offers crisis housing and debt assistance. The Web site contains a state-by-state searchable database of local organizations that provide similar services.

Health Advocate
www.healthadvocate.com
1 (866) 695-8622
The Health Advocate offers many of the same services as the Center for Patient Partnerships and is normally available through your health plan. However, Health Advocate will review individual cases for an hourly fee.

Healthcare Navigation, LLC
www.healthcarenavigation.com

1 (203) 655-1156
Healthcare Navigation focuses its advocacy services on
billing and insurance issues, and does not offer medical advice or help in choosing doctors. The service is based on an
hourly fee.

Among the most expensive ways to find a doctor are "personal
patient advocate services," which for a substantial fee will research the top specialists for you, handle your appointment, test,
and insurance paperwork, and even help you bypass a doctor's
waiting list. One of the best-known companies in this group is
Pinnacle Care International [www.pinnaclecare.com; 1 (866) 752-
1712].

In the Hospital

Many conditions that even a few years ago required extensive
hospitalization are handled on an outpatient basis now, which
means that if you are in the hospital, you are probably pretty
sick.

Based on my experience and the recommendations of the
people I interviewed (including the physicians and nurses), if at
all possible, you should try to have a family member or friend
with you at all times except possibly at night. That is an organizational challenge that many of us are not up for. If you or your
loved one is very ill, however, it is the best course. Between the
short staffing at many hospitals and the high prevalence of medical errors, it is worth trying to do this.

Hospitals have other professional resources that may be very
helpful to you, whether or not you are alone:

NURSES
Floor nurses are the ones who are there all the time and have seen
minute-by-minute ups and downs of your condition many times
before. They are skilled and educated and are an invaluable resource, although they are probably very busy. They know how
things get done and can help you figure out what is going on.
Chances are, however, they won't have a lot of time to chat and

may have many patients who are acutely ill, so collect your concerns for when you catch them rather than buzzing around asking questions three or four times an hour. You may want to introduce yourself to the *nurse manager* who is in charge of your floor or unit, if you think you might be around for more than a couple days.

Clinical nurse specialists have become an important fixture of many hospital units, and they are pure gold. Ask if there is one assigned to your unit or if there is one who specializes in your disease working at the hospital.

Clinical nurse specialists are masters–level experts trained in managing the transitions in health and life brought on by serious medical conditions. They can help you understand the impact and progression of the disease and the effects of the treatment, help you anticipate what might happen next, and explain the practical aspects of tests and their meaning.

This is not to say, of course, that your physician couldn't tell you most of these things, should she or he have time, but your doctor's focus is generally more on treating the disease, whereas the clinical nurse specialist's focus is on you and what you need to participate fully in your care.

MEDICAL SOCIAL WORKER

The job of medical social workers is to connect you with the information and resources that you need in order to move on to the next stage of your care. "For example," said Cheryl Dunlop, a medical social worker in Little Rock, Arkansas, "if the referral comes from oncology and someone is going to get radiation and chemotherapy, we have booklets and videos on treatment, we can answer questions and we have a wig room and donated cosmetics and can work with them on a living will.

"If they have had a stroke, we evaluate to see if they need acute rehabilitation or a nursing home. It is a huge decision to take away someone's independence like this, so we try not to, which means that we work to get all the equipment into the home, get someone to be there twenty–four hours a day, and arrange the social systems that are needed, including figuring out the disability and workman's compensation and insurance and getting started applying for SSI and Medicaid.

"But sometimes medical social work can also just be getting the family vouchers for the cafeteria."

Your doctor may have already asked a social worker to come see you, but if not, you may need to ask your physician or the hospitalist to write an order for the social worker to come visit you if you feel you need help with the practical arrangements of moving out of the hospital.

PATIENT NAVIGATOR

Patient navigators are most often available through hospitals for their patients, especially those who have public insurance such as Medicaid, nonnative speakers, and people with disabilities. Sometimes these navigators are part of the hospital's volunteer force and occasionally they are part of a federal program. The Patient Navigator Act, passed in 2005, makes money available for new navigator programs run by the Indian Health Service, the Office of Rural Health Policy, and the National Cancer Institute. The National Cancer Institute has been testing patient navigator programs at several sites around the country since the 1990s. Some nonprofit organizations fund navigator programs at hospitals around the country, as the Breast Cancer Research Foundation does for several hospitals in New York City.

Patient navigators can be nurses or doctors, but often they are social workers or even other patients who had much experience dealing with a particular diagnosis and the worries and paperwork that come along for the ride. Depending on their background, navigators can help you schedule appointments with specialists, explain your test results and walk you through your options for treatment, check into billing problems, refer you to counseling, or just listen to your concerns with an ear toward how they can help. In many cases, patient navigators will seek you out after your diagnosis or treatment at a hospital to make sure you get the proper follow-up care and come to all your next appointments. Patient navigators work especially with patients who have no insurance, those who rarely see a doctor and may not be familiar with the health-care system, and those who speak a language other than English.

The best way to find a navigator in your community is to check with your local hospital, preferably a hospital where you will be receiving treatment if necessary. In most cases, navigator services are free of charge.

For a referral to a patient navigator that is not necessarily associated with a hospital, you can check out some of the voluntary health organizations such as the American Cancer Society [1 (800) ACS-2345] for information on navigators in your area (see appendix G for other nonprofit organizations). Navigators recommended by ACS and others are usually less helpful for specific billing and appointment information and more useful for finding general resources for your condition in your area and connecting you to other support professionals.

CLERGY

If you are in the hospital near your home and are connected to a faith community, a representative of that community may come see you. In many hospitals, however, there are also hospital chaplains who make the rounds to see patients. You probably noticed that when you were admitted to the hospital, you were asked to check a box indicating your religious preference.

As someone who holds my faith pretty close to my vest, I have been testy about these visits, which seem to occur regardless of which box I check. The last thing I want when I am sick is someone prying into that part of my life.

But in talking with others, I've found that I am the exception: many of the people I talked to (and their families) really valued the presence of someone who was not part of the worried community of loved ones who had the time to listen to what was going on. A couple of people said they talked about fears they couldn't share with their families. Another said the chaplain was able to mediate some tense family disputes and help everyone calm down.

The charge of health-care chaplains is not to proselytize but rather to be present, to hold your hand to validate your feelings, and to talk about whatever you want to talk about, whether it is that you feel abandoned by God or that you don't know how to tell your mother you are so ill.

If you would welcome a visit by the chaplain and none has appeared, you should be able to request one by calling the chaplain's office if there is one, or by asking the nurse how to arrange to be seen by a member of the clergy. Every institution will have this service available in some form appropriate to patients of any religion.

CONSULTATION–LIAISON PSYCHIATRIST

If you or your loved one is overwhelmed by emotions and is unable to sleep, to stop crying, or to stop raging, or if your loved one has withdrawn into himself and is unwilling to communicate or cooperate with treatment, you may want to request a consultation from a psychiatrist.

Consultation–liaison psychiatrists are psychiatrists who specialize in treating people with medical illness within hospitals. They are accustomed to working with people who have received devastating diagnoses. They have expertise not only in the emotional and cognitive side effects of medication, but also in prescribing antianxiety medication, for example, that won't have an adverse interaction with the medication you are already taking. Your physician, the hospitalist, or the nurse manager can help you get this kind of help.

PATIENT ADVOCATE

One of the good things about hospitals being run as businesses is that they increasingly are concerned about "customer" satisfaction and often have designated staff whose job it is to address complaints. There should be a telephone number for you to call in the hospital directory.

If you have questions about the care you have been receiving, if you feel that your physician has not been attending to your care, if you are concerned that an error has been made in your care, call that number. Ask to see someone in your room that same day, tell him or her your concerns and indicate that you are willing to work with him or her to solve this problem immediately. Don't wait until you fill out the rating form as you leave the hospital to make your complaint known. Think of your complaint as an opportunity to make things better.

Alternatively, you can call the complaint number at the Joint Commission on Accreditation of Healthcare Organizations (www.jointcommission.org/GeneralPublic/Complaint/default.htm) or your state licensing board (usually located in the state department of health).

Voluntary and Nonprofit Organizations

T HIS APPENDIX LISTS only a few of the nonprofit, voluntary organizations that can help you with information about your disease, treatment, financial and insurance aid, mental health counseling, and generally living with your condition. These voluntary organizations, such as the American Cancer Society, and the American Heart Association, range in size and services, but in general they are associations that have come together for a specific cause, such as raising money for disease research or providing health information to people with a specific disease. Nonprofit organizations reinvest any money they make back into their services and programs. The ".org" suffix at the end of Web site addresses indicates that an organization is a nonprofit.

Before reading on, it's good to remember a few tips about seeking information from hotlines and Web sites.

Telephone Help Lines

Telephone help lines are one of the most valuable free services available to people with a new serious diagnosis. There are many of them, however, and they offer different kinds of help, so it is a good idea to figure out what you want before you call and ask if they can help you—and if not, if they know of a telephone service that can.

The other key to making good use of a telephone service is— if you have been satisfied with your conversation—to ask if you can have your operator's personal extension and call back with additional questions.

Telephone help lines are sponsored by health plans, employers, nonprofit disease organizations, and the government.

The three main kinds of help such telephone lines offer are:

1. *Access to good information*

The quintessential telephone line for information is the U.S. Government's 1 (800) 4–CANCER from the National Cancer Institute. It is staffed by trained operators who are not necessarily medical professionals, but who can offer information about your condition, available treatments, clinical trials, and disease statistics. They cannot offer individual medical advice or counseling. After discussing what you need to know, they may send you booklets that provide more information or refer you to their extensive Web site.

2. *Advice about self care and health emergencies*

These telephone lines are not open to the public generally, but you may have access to one that is sponsored by your health plan or employer. If so, you will find the number in the description of your benefits. Such lines are usually staffed by nurses. Their purpose is to help to distinguish between those symptoms and situations that are serious and need immediate medical attention, those that can wait to see a doctor until tomorrow, and those you can care for yourself. Anyone who has deliberated about whether a cut is serious enough to require stitches can appreciate the value of having twenty-four-hour access to this kind of advice. If your condition is fragile or you have a rare disease, advice nurses may not be the best match for you, as they tend to have more expertise in responding to common disorders and accidents.

3. *Health coaching*

Some telephone help lines—also those offered through health plans and employers—offer access to a health coach. A health coach will help you:

— Find out what you need to know about your condition

— Establish a frame of reference, a way to think about what is going on

— Focus on the next decision you need to make

— Make a plan of action

— Practice your next conversation with your doctor

Online Support: Chat Rooms, Discussion Groups, Message Boards

Many Web sites associated with nonprofit groups feature Internet chat rooms, discussion groups, or message boards that focus on specific issues (enrolling in clinical trials, for instance) or general questions (such as, "Does the nausea ever go away on this medication?"). Many patients find these resources invaluable, because they connect them with a community of people going through the same ups and downs and or lead them to different resources that they might not otherwise find.

The quality of these resources varies, however, depending on how the site organizes and monitors its online groups. Groups may be monitored infrequently to remove inappropriate posts and to keep participants civil, but some sites allow a free-for-all among participants that can be unnerving to first-time users. Other sites offer chats and support groups that are led by a professional monitor, including doctors, counselors, or financial managers. As with all Internet resources, it's good to check out who's behind the information you read.

Online Tips

- Many nonprofit groups offer their materials or hotline advice in Spanish and occasionally in other languages.

- National disease organizations, such as the American Cancer Society and the National Multiple Sclerosis Society, have local chapters all around the country that can be an excellent resource for you after checking out what the national organization has to offer. Local chapters can often give out doctor referrals and information on local programs and events that national organizations aren't willing or able to provide.

Disease-Specific Organizations

CANCER

American Cancer Society
www.cancer.org

1 (800) ACS-2345 (24 hours, 7 days a week, toll-free)
The ACS Web site contains information on cancer, survival statistics, treatment options, and ways to connect with cancer survivor online communities and local support groups. The site also features a free matching service for finding clinical trials in your area, online treatment decision tools, and a database of doctors and hospitals around the country. On the twenty-four-hour hotline, you can speak with cancer information specialists, people trained to answer a variety of questions about cancer, your insurance, and employment rights after a diagnosis and general questions about ACS services and events. They will also mail pamphlets on most topics covered by the Web site. These specialists cannot give medical advice, provide mental health support or find a doctor for you over the phone.

Cancer Care
www.cancercare.org
1 (800) 813-4673 (toll-free)
This nonprofit Web site offers some information on the specific and free counseling the organization provides to cancer patients and their families, including face-to-face and telephone support groups. The hotline is staffed by oncology social workers who can answer questions about your disease, treatment, financial assistance, insurance, and work issues.

Steve Dunn's Cancer Guide
http://cancerguide.org
Steve Dunn, a kidney cancer patient who died in August 2005, created an extensive Web site that doesn't have information about specific cancers but focuses instead on how to research your treatment options, learning what questions to ask your doctors, and coping with financial and practical aspects of confronting cancer. The site also contains detailed strategies for finding and enrolling in clinical trials.

People Living with Cancer
www.plwc.org
The PLWC Web site is a service of the American Society of Clinical Oncologists. The site contains extensive information on eighty-five different types of cancers, articles on coping

with the disease, a primer on clinical trials and links to clinical trial databases, and a searchable national database of oncologists who are ASCO members. The site does not have a hotline service.

Association of Cancer Online Resources (ACOR)
www.acor.org
ACOR is a clearinghouse site of online communities (mailing lists, support groups, hosted Web sites) specifically for people coping with cancer. The extensive group of mailing lists includes special lists for specific types of cancer, as well as more general issues such as survivorship, financial planning, and caregiving. The lists are free and unmoderated, but commercial activities such as pitching cancer drugs, are forbidden.

HEART DISEASE

American Heart Association
www.americanheart.org
1 (800) 242-8721 (24 hours, 7 days a week, toll-free)
The AHA Web site contains information on a variety of heart diseases and an online treatment decision tool. At the twenty-four-hour hotline, trained operators can answer your questions about any information contained on the Web site and mail pamphlets offered on almost any topic covered by the Web site. The operators cannot give medical advice, refer you to doctors in your area, or provide mental health support.

STROKE

American Stroke Association
www.strokeassociation.org
1 (888) 478-7653 (24 hours, 7 days a week, toll-free)
The ASA Web site has medical information about stroke, a list of Web sites that provide more information on financial aid for stroke medications and a database of doctors, hospitals, and rehabilitation centers that have been recognized for quality care of stroke patients by organizations like the

National Committee for Quality Assurance (see chapter 4 and appendix C). Services provided at the twenty-four-hour hotline are similar to those offered by the American Heart Association hotline.

LUNG DISEASE

American Lung Association
www.lungusa.org/
1 (800) 548-8252 (toll-free)
The American Lung Association Web site contains general information about diseases including lung cancer, emphysema, and chronic obstructive pulmonary disease (COPD). The site also has online decision treatment tools for a number of conditions. The Association's hotline is staffed by registered nurses and respiratory therapists who can answer questions about your disease, refer you to a doctor in your area and counsel you on insurance, medication, and case management problems.

Lung Cancer Online Foundation
www.lungcanceronline.org
The Lung Cancer Online Web site is a guide to Web sites on all topics related to lung cancer, from general information about the disease to treatment options, doctor searches, and support groups. The foundation does not run a hotline service.

ALZHEIMER'S DISEASE

Alzheimer's Association
www.alz.org/
1 (800) 272-3900 (24 hours, 7 days a week, toll-free)
The Alzheimer's Association Web site has information about the disease, including treatments and statistics, help for caregivers, information on Medicare and Medicaid insurance, a list of current clinical trials, and the ability to search the organization's extensive Alzheimer's library. (The librarians will make photocopies of any article for $10.) The twenty-four-hour hotline is staffed by both trained operators who can assist you with general questions about the disease, treatment,

insurance and financial issues, and other information on the Web site. The hotline can also connect you with a clinician who can give you specific personalized advice using decision-making treatment tools, as well as answer care-givers' questions.

MULTIPLE SCLEROSIS
National Multiple Sclerosis Society
www.nationalmssociety.org
1 (800) 344-4867
The National Multiple Sclerosis Society has a fifty-state net-work of chapters that offer employment counseling, family programs, volunteer opportunities, and information about advocacy. The national office sponsors an elegant, easy-to-use Web site that includes information and Web casts about the disease, its treatment, and advice about finding good health care generally and at affiliated treatment facilities. You can subscribe to the society's periodicals and download pamphlets, as well as browse through the library online. The society's 800 telephone number connects you directly to the chapter nearest to you.

PARKINSON'S DISEASE
National Parkinson's Foundation
www.parkinson.org
1 (800)327-4545 (toll-free)

American Parkinson Disease Association Inc.
www.apdaparkinson.org/
1 (800) 223-2732 (toll-free)
Web sites for these two Parkinson's organizations contain general and limited information on the disease and treat-ment. The National Parkinson's Foundation site has an online library of articles that can be downloaded free. The hotlines for both organizations do not provide medical advice, mental health counseling, or doctor referrals. However, each Web site and hotline can give you contact information for local chap-ters that may help you find some of these services.

ALS

The ALS Association
www.alsa.org/
1 (800) 782-4747
The ALS (amyotrophic lateral sclerosis) Web site contains
general information about the disease, an order form for free
pamphlets and videos on a variety of topics, and links to
other organizations that may help you with financial or legal
questions related to your treatment. The site also contains a
useful guide to understanding your Medicare eligibility. Operators at the hotline can answer questions about information found on the Web site, take orders for pamphlets and
videos, and offer doctor referrals in your area. They cannot
give medical advice or mental health counseling.

LUPUS

Lupus Foundation of America
www.lupus.org
1 (202) 349-1155 (8:30 AM–5 PM eastern standard time,
Monday–Friday)
The LFA Web site provides a good starting point to learn the
basics about lupus, its diagnosis, and its treatment. You can
use the NLM interactive tutorial to get the basics and explore
the Web site for more in-depth information, such as finding
the nearest chapter. Chapters provide support groups, information about local and regional services, and sponsor fund-
raising events. The foundation does not support a telephone
hotline, but provides an information request line in English
(1–800–558–0121) and in Spanish (1–800–558–0231). You can get
a referral to a health educator or leave your name and address to be sent introductory materials.

DIABETES

American Diabetes Association
www.diabetes.org
1 (800) DIABETES (1–800–342–2383). Monday–Friday, 8:30
AM–8 PM eastern standard time
The American Diabetes Association has an easy-to-use Web

site packed with information. Click on "Newly Diagnosed" and the site will walk you through the disease and its management in a straightforward and practical way. Like many of the voluntary health organizations, the ADA Web site contains a wealth of information for the public and professionals with a range of interests, from prevention to management and treatment. ADA also produces and collects materials about diabetes for different groups: children, Asian Pacific Islanders, African Americans, Latinos, Native Americans, people with Type 1 or Type 2, adolescents, etc. If you prefer not to use the Web site, call the 800 number and discuss the information you think would be helpful or ask them to identify the closest chapter.

HIV/AIDS

There are many nonprofit organizations focused on HIV/AIDS, but a good place to start looking for information on the disease, treatments, medication, lifestyle changes, insurance, financial aid, and workplace legal issues is The Body, (www.thebody.com), a clearinghouse Web site that draws information from over one hundred nonprofit and other organizations, and that offers a list of state HIV/AIDS hotlines.

Centers for Disease Control and Prevention Hotline
1 (800) CDC-INFO ((24 hours, 7 days a week, toll-free)
Operators at the CDC hotline can give you general information about HIV infection and AIDS as well as refer you to local hotlines, clinics, counseling, and support groups. They do not provide mental health counseling or specific doctor referrals.

AIDS.org
(www.aids.org/info/hotlines.html) Another source for state hotlines. Hours and services vary, but most of them offer general information about the disease and can refer you to local clinics and counseling services.

Project Inform National Hotline
1 (800) 822-7422 (toll-free)

The Project Inform national hotline offers advice on HIV/AIDS medication and blood work, referrals to local clinics, and counseling and pamphlets on different topics related to treatment and living with the disease.

OTHER SERVICES

American Self-Help Group Clearinghouse—Self-Help Group Sourcebook Online
www.mentalhelp.net/selfhelp/
This online sourcebook contains links to and contact information for over 100 self-help groups for a variety of diseases, from AIDS and heart disease to rare genetic disorders. The site also contains a list of toll-free numbers for self-help groups around the country.

Veterans Administration (VA)
1 (877) 222-8387 (toll-free)
www1.va.gov/Health_Benefits/
Not technically a nonprofit group, the Veterans Administration has a wealth of health information and programs available to veterans throughout the country. If you are eligible for these services, you may want to check out their Web site or call their hotline to find out more about the available programs. The VA offers insurance and financial assistance, support through national chaplains' network and social work services, and special programs for patients with cancer, HIV/AIDS, diabetes, blindness, kidney disease, and injuries.

Financial Help and Estate Planning

Financial Planning

A<small>S MANY PATIENTS HAVE FOUND</small>, a serious illness can quickly deplete your financial resources, or, at the very least, deplete your ability and willingness to plan for your financial future. But it's important to keep up with your finances at this time, for several reasons. You need to make sure you have as much money as you can find to pay for whatever treatments you might need. You need to ensure that you and your family can live comfortably while you might be out of work for a while. Even if you're the one who normally handles the family checkbook or makes the financial decisions for the family, your skills might not be up to the long-term financial planning that's necessary in the face of a serious illness. Your financial outlook may change as well; you're not saving for the rainy day anymore, you're spending that rainy-day budget.

Financial planners can evaluate your budget, suggest changes in your investments, set up a bill payment plan, and help you with tax and insurance questions. There are several kinds of professionals who can give you this type of advice, from certified public accountants to certified financial planners. If possible, look for someone who has had experience in handling finances for other patients like you. Organizations such as the American Cancer Society can help you find an experienced professional (you can request the pamphlet "How to Find a Financial Professional Sensitive to Cancer Issues" using their hotline or on their Web site) through your local chapter. If you belong to a support group, people in the group may also be able to give you some good references.

Other places to look for a certified financial planner include:

Certified Financial Planner Board of Standards, Inc.
1 (888) 237-6275
www.cfp.net/

The Financial Planning Association
1 (800) 322-4237
www.fpanet.org/public/index.cfm

The National Association of Personal Financial Planners
1 (800) 366-2732
www.napfa.org/index2.htm

Society of Financial Service Professionals
1 (888) 243-2258
www.financialpro.org/Consumer/find.cfm

Financial, Insurance, and Legal Aid
Nonprofit Services

For general financial, insurance, and legal aid help, check the nonprofit resources below. They offer financial planning assistance for free or for a small fee. Other good places to look for this kind of help are local religious and cultural organizations, which can sometimes provide services ranging from financial assistance, legal advice, and even transportation to your doctor's office or other critical appointments.

National Endowment for Financial Education
www.nefe.org/pages/collaborative.html
This nonprofit group specializes in personal finance education. NEFE maintains a list of links to other Web materials and Web sites from disease organizations that specifically discuss financial and insurance information related to coping with a serious illness.

Consolidated Credit Counseling Services Inc.
www.consolidatedcredit.org/
1 (800) 320-9929 (toll-free)
This nonprofit organization can counsel you regarding your financial situation, including any nonmedical expenses or

debts, and set up a special payment plan for you that re-
duces your number of monthly bills. The organization
charges a small processing fee for the payment services, and
you must have at least $2,000 in debt to qualify for the
program.

The Center for Patient Partnerships at the University of
Wisconsin
www.law.wisc.edu/patientadvocacy/
The center offers help in understanding your diagnosis, solving insurance snarls and making sense of medical bills,
searching for a second opinion, and determining your eligibility for federal and state benefit programs for people with
chronic or life–threatening illnesses all across the country.
The service is free of charge.

Patient Advocate Foundation
www.patientadvocate.org
1 (800) 532–5274
The Patient Advocate Foundation is a nonprofit organization
that can work with insurers, creditors, and employers on
coverage appeals, employee benefits, and bill payment. The
foundation also offers crisis housing and debt assistance. The
Web site contains a state–by–state searchable database of
local organizations that provide similar services.

Medicare Rights Center
www.medicarerights.org
The Medicare Rights Center offers free information and
counseling to people with Medicare coverage. Most of the information is available on their Web site, but the Center does
run special hotlines with limited hours for patients using
Medicare through an HMO and Medicare patients in New
York State. The Web site also contains an extensive list of toll-
free numbers for Medicare patients to call in each state.

Catastrophic Health Planners
410–861–8969
www.chp1.org
The mission of Catastrophic Health Planners is to insure that
people and families facing a catastrophic health event can

make informed decisions regarding issues that affect their quality of life. This organization offers a wide range of advice about financial legal matters, insurance options, medical alternatives, Social Security and disability information, and support. It provides free educational development, support, and referral services to patients and families facing a devastating diagnosis.

Cancer and Careers
www.cancerandcareers.org/resources/
The Cancer and Careers Web site offers a large set of links to legal, financial and insurance information in its Resource Database. Some of the information is specific to certain states such as California and New York, but many of the links contain general information.

Kaiser Family Foundation
1 (202) 347-5270
www.kff.org/consumerguide/7350.cfm
The Kaiser Family Foundation published a consumer guide to handling health insurance disputes with your employer or health-care plan. The guide is regularly updated and is available for free. It does not cover disputes with Medicare or Medicaid, however.

Partnership for Prescription Assistance
www.pparx.org
1 (888) 477-2669
This program is a clearinghouse for more than 475 public and private programs that help patients without prescription coverage get the medicine they need for free or nearly free. You can search for programs that cover your medicines and download application forms for some programs on the Web site, or request information over the phone at the toll-free number.

NeedyMeds
www.needymeds.com/
Provides a similar service to Partnership for Prescription Assistance.

Public Support (Medicare, Medicaid, Social Security Disability Insurance)

If you have a catastrophic illness and know that it will push you beyond your means, you may want to start the process to apply for public support. You may already be enrolled in these programs and want to learn how to make further advantage of what they offer. Or you may not realize that your condition allows you to enroll in programs such as Medicare, which you might have thought was out of reach at your age. Below are the three major types of government health insurance programs. There is a lot of paperwork and months–long lead time to enroll in these programs, so even if you're only thinking about enrolling, it might be worth a few minutes to check out the possibilities now.

Medicare
www.medicare.gov/default.asp
1 (800) MEDICARE (24 hours a day/ 7 days a week)
Medicare is a federal health insurance program for citizens and permanent residents of the United States age sixty-five and older. Generally, you are eligible for Medicare if you fall into this category, although there are conditions related to how long you have worked in Medicare–covered employment during your or your spouse's life and length of residency requirements that affect which parts of the Medicare program you must pay for. You can also qualify for coverage if you are younger than sixty-five but have permanent kidney failure requiring dialysis or a transplant, if you have been diagnosed with amyotrophic lateral sclerosis (ALS), or if you have been receiving Social Security Disability Insurance for more than twenty-four months (see pages 255–256). For most eligible enrollees, Medicare Part A (hospital insurance) is free, but you must pay a monthly premium for Medicare Part B (medical insurance that covers doctors' visits and other outpatient services.) In 2006, Part D, a prescription drug benefit administered through private health plans was added to the Medicare lineup.

If you are getting Social Security benefits when you turn age sixty-five, you will automatically be enrolled in Medicare Parts A and B. If you are not getting Social Security at age sixty-five, or if you are enrolling at another time in your life, you should allow at least three months for processing of your application and enrollment in the program.

For more information on enrollment and eligibility, you can call the hotline number (English and Spanish-speaking representatives are available) or go the Web site listed above. A quick warning: the Medicare Web site is chock full of information and experiences a heavy volume of traffic each day, so navigating the site can be slow and frustrating if you're looking for answers to a specific question. Another good place to look for quick, basic information on Medicare is the nonprofit group Medicare Rights Center (see page 252).

Medicaid
www.cms.hhs.gov/medicaid/consumer.asp
1 (877) 267-2323
Medicaid is a public health insurance program that is run as a partnership between federal and individual state governments. In general, Medicaid offers health coverage to several groups of people with low income and few resources such as your own home. People who are blind or disabled and have a low income are some of Medicaid's main beneficiaries. The program does not pay money directly to you, but rather pays money out to your doctors. (You may have to make a small copayment in some instances.) Medicaid benefits and eligibility can vary from state to state. The lag time between enrollment and full benefits also varies, but three months is a good rule of thumb here, too.

For more information on enrollment and eligibility, it's best to contact your state Medicaid program directly. The phone number above will connect you with the federal Centers for Medicare and Medicaid Services, who can offer you general information about Medicaid. This information, along with direct contact information for each state, is also located on the Web site above.

Social Security Disability Insurance/ Supplemental Security Income Program
www.ssa.gov/d&s1.htm
1 (800) 772-1213

These two programs, administered by the Social Security Administration, are the largest federal disability assistance programs. *Social Security Disability Insurance* pays monthly cash benefits to a person who is disabled (or to some members of their immediate family), under age sixty-five and who has not been able to work for a year or more due to their disability. The idea here is that the benefits will continue until you are able to go back to work on a regular basis, or until you turn sixty-five and the benefits turn into retirement benefits. To participate in this program, you must have worked in jobs covered by Social Security for a certain period in recent years. The *Supplemental Security Income* (SSI) program makes monthly cash payments to people who are aged (age sixty-five or older), blind, or disabled, and who have a low income. The payment can be used for essentials such as food, clothing, and housing.

It takes three to five months to process disability claims, and paperwork from your former employers and your physicians, as well as tax information, are necessary to apply to both programs. The phone number and Web site, again, can direct you to more specific eligibility and enrollment information.

Advance Directives, Living Wills, and Medical Power of Attorney

These documents spell out your wishes for your medical care when you are incapacitated and unable to make your preferences known. Many people think these documents become important only at the end of life or in dire situations such as irreversible brain damage or coma, but you can use an advance directive, for instance, to specify what kinds of treatments you do not want under any circumstances during the course of your care.

An *advance directive* is any legal document in which you give instructions about your health care that should be followed when you are unable to speak for yourself. A *living will* is a type of advance directive that usually refers to your wishes about life-sustaining treatments when you are terminally ill. *Medical Power of Attorney*, *Health-Care Power of Attorney* or *Health-Care Proxy* are terms that refer the legal rights you give to someone you choose who will make medical treatment decisions for you if you can't make them yourself.

Everyone, regardless of how healthy, should consider drawing up an advance directive of some kind. Your directive should contain information that is especially important to you, taking into account your family's needs and your personal and spiritual beliefs about medical treatment. For instance, you may ask for a "do-not-resuscitate" order that keeps hospital staff from giving you CPR in the event that your heart stops or you stop breathing. Or, you may want to ask for painkiller medication even after all other treatments have been stopped. Similarly, you can appoint a person to have medical power of attorney, but spell out exactly what that person can and cannot do.

The laws regarding advance directives vary from state to state. If you divide your time between two states, create a separate document for each state, appointing a person appropriate to each jurisdiction to be your proxy (could be the same person). In general, it's important to put your wishes down in writing, to get legal witnesses for your document and to be as specific as possible in terms of treatment and identifying those who can and cannot speak for you. You can change your advance directive at any time.

After you have written your advance directives and had them notarized, you should make several copies of the document. One should be kept in a secure place that your family members are familiar with, such as a household safe. You should give a copy to the person you have asked to have medical power of attorney and his or her backup, if there is someone in that position and any other members of your family who you think might be called if there is a medical emergency. You should also take copies to the hospital if you will be admitted for treatment, so that your physicians are aware of your wishes.

Many hospitals now provide a short version of an advance directive document to patients when they are admitted to the hospital. In many cases, these documents simply spell out some basic decisions ("do you want to be resuscitated in the event of…") and ask for your signature. Remember: you do *not* have to sign a hospital's advance directive form to receive care.

If you have a personal attorney or access to legal services already, you may want to draw up your advance directive with professionals you already know. If not, you may want to speak to an attorney with specific expertise.

National Academy of Elder Law Attorneys
http://naela.org
This is an organization of lawyers with interest, training, and experience in advance directives and living wills. They can be helpful in understanding the legal requirements of your state. The Web site includes a referral service.

There are several resources available to learn more about advance directives, legal requirements in your state and forms that can guide you in creating the specific document:

The American Bar Association—Commission on Law and Aging
http://abanet.org/aging
1 (202) 662-8690
The ABA offers several health-care decision tools on its Web site, including a consumer's toolkit for advance health-care planning and a pamphlet specifically on advance directives that includes a sample form.

Aging with Dignity—Five Wishes Advance Directive
www.agingwithdignity.org/5wishes.html
1 (888) 594-7437
This popular advance directive from the nonprofit organization Aging with Dignity walks you through preparing a directive that can include your treatment preferences, medical power of attorney, how you want to be treated in the hospital apart from your medical treatment, and how you might want to be remembered in the event of your death. The form and directions cost $5 and can be ordered online or over the phone.

The Medical Directive
www.medicaldirective.org
This nonprofit organization offers a comprehensive living will form that was first published in the *Journal of the American Medical Association*. The document asks questions regarding six different scenarios such as coma, and asks you to check off what kinds of treatment you would find acceptable un-

der each scenario. The form costs $15 and can be ordered online only or through the mail (mailing address is at the Web site).

Caring Connections
www.caringinfo.org
1 (800) 658–8898
Caring Connections, a service of the National Hospice and Palliative Care Organization, offers information on advance directives, including state-specific directive forms and legal requirements. You can get this information for free through their Web site or by calling their hotline.

U.S. Living Will Registry
www.uslivingwillregistry.com
1 (800) 548–9455
The Living Will Registry is a for-profit company that will store your advance directive electronically in a database where your health-care providers can access it at any time. Storage is free to individuals who register their directive through health-care providers who have agreed to be members in the service. You can call the hotline above or check out the Web site to see if there are any members in your area.

The following Web sites offer more information about advance directives:

MedlinePlus
"Advance Directives"
www.nlm.nih.gov/medlineplus./advancedirectives.html

WebMD—"Planning for Incapacity: Legal Issues of Caregiving"
http://my.webmd.com/content/article/45/4041_111?z=4041_30

American Academy of Family Physicians—"Advance Directives and Do Not Resuscitate Orders"
http://familydoctor.org/003.xml

Some things just can't be done alone.

Responding to a devastating diagnosis is one of them.

I have weathered the storm of each of my own with the unwavering love and support of my beloved husband, Richard Sloan; my parents, Ellie and Larry Gruman; my brothers, Pete, Paul, and Jep Gruman; my co-workers Rena Convissor, Becky Ham, who also conducted the research for this book, Ira Allen, Barbara Krimgold, David Torresen; my friends and my colleagues all over the world. Words cannot capture my gratitude to them.

Writing a book about responding to a devastating diagnosis is another endeavor best undertaken with others.

I have been privileged to be able to draw on the expertise and experiences of the following people, each of whom contributed to this project out of a sense of solidarity with those who will read it. Thank you.

Donna Abelli, Ron Abeles, Nancy Adler, Michelle Alexander, Diane Amato, Nancy Anderson, Dr. Karen Antman, Diane Archer, Dr. Deborah Axelrod, Dr. Janet Baradell, Dr. Jeremiah Barondess, Dr. John Bascom, Clara Behar, Barbara Bejoian, Dr. Lawrence Bergner, Linda Bergthold, Barbara Berkman, Cathy Blackburn, Andy Burness, Dorothy Gulbenkian Blaney, Diane Blum, Dr. Jeremy Boal, Nora Boustany, Rosie Boustany, Dr. Matt Budd, Nancy Breen, Dr. William Breitbart, Joseph Califano, Dr. Ned Cassem, Dr. Rita Charon, Thomas Chirikos, Dr. Carolyn Clancy, Connie Clark, Richard Clark, Dr. Dexanne Clohan, Dr. E. Dale Collins, Nancy Colon, Dr. James Cooper, Ilene Clucas, Carol Cronin, Sue Curry, Karina Davidson, Connie Davis, Regina Davis, Gary Deimling, Dr. Allan Deitrich, Dr. Bruce Doblin, Christina Donawa, Carol Dougherty, Meryl Doxer, Cheryl Dunlop, Joann Eckstut, Polly Eddy, Michal Ehlman, Allan Erickson, Lynn Etheredge, Brock Evans, Dr. Claire Fagin, Mindy Fast, David Feffer, Kathy Fennelly, Joel Fleishman, Dr. Andrew Fishman, Susan Fitzpatrick, Jack Fowler, Dan Fox, Lina Fruzzetti, Jonathan Fuchs, Meg Gaines, Kate Gibson, Elinor Ginzler, Hope Gleicher, Dr. Jerry Glicklich, Tom Glynn, Dr. Marthe Gold,

Janlori Goldman, Barbara Goldsmith, Catherine Gordon, Ken Gorfinkle, Rob Gould, Loretta Graf, Donna Grande, Janet Green, Vartan Gregorian, Ellen Gritz, Dr. Jerome Groopman, Bernard Gross, Joe Hafey, Elli Hall, George Handzo, T. George Harris, Brian Hawkins, Veronica Hearst, Richard Heffner, Clara Hernandez, Judy Hibbard, Dr. Jimmie Holland, Sandra Horning, Eliana Horta, Margot Hover, Marcia Hurst, Alice Ilchman, Charles Inlander, David Introcaso, Howard Isenstein, Jim Jaffe, Dorothy Jeffress, Dr. Roger Johns, Dr. David Johnson, Jackie Johnson, Melissa Johnson, Stan Jones, Judy Miller Jones, Lisa Jorgenson, Dr. Sarah Kagan, Dr. Doug Kamerow, Wendy Katkin, Ruth Katz, Arthur Kelly, Elizabeth Kelly, Larry Kessler, Linda King, Margaret Kirk, Dan Kohrman, Beth Kosiak, Jean Kraemer, Dr. Robert Krasner, Fred Krimgold, Clyde Laney, Pauline Lapin, Ray Lawrence, Margaret Lazar, Rick Lee, Susan Leigh, Eleanor Lerman, Dr. Robert Levine, Susan Edgeman–Levitan, Don Liss, Maral Markarian, Margaret Mahoney, Susan Margolies, Elizabeth McCormack, Gaynor McCown, Shelley McKaye, Jim McNaughton, Dr. Al Mulley, Dr. Robert Melton, Maria Menocal, Michael Millenson, Suzanne Miller, Catherine Monk, Dr. David Muller, Dr. Mary Mundinger, MaryAnn Napoli, Ted Nash, Dr. David Nathan, Ron Nofsinger, Dr. Afaf Meleis, Kathy O'Connell, Annette O'Connor, Catherine O'Neill, Akos Oster, Ana Palacio, Anne Pashby, Mike Pertschuk, Mario Pitchon, Todd Plitt, Kari Plotsky, Dr. William Popick, Ellen Pryga, Diane Quale, Marge Ramey, Dr. Paula Rauch, Donna Regenstreif, Corrine Reider, Paula Reiger, Marilyn Richards, Andrew Robinson, Elizabeth Rohatyn, Betty Rollin, William Rosenberg, Dr. John Rowe, Julia Rowland, Karin Rush–Monroe, Phyllis Saltzman, Dr. Steve Schoenbaum, Dr. Larry Schulman, Don Schumacher, Malcolm Schwartz, Ann Seger, Josh Seidman, Dr. Steve Shea, Dr. Deborah Schrag, Dr. Teresa Schrader, Dr. Suzanne Smith, Anna Sofaer, Shoshanna Sofaer, Christina Spellman, Dr. David Spiegel, Donna Sperry, Cohevet Spiro, Eshel Spiro, Dr. Kurt Stange, Ellen Stover, Heidi Stolp, Dr. Hugh Straley, Wendy Strothman, Dr. Neville Strumpf, Roxie Sudjian, Dr. Eileen Marx Sullivan, Dr. Owen Surman, Drita Taraila, Linda Tarr–Whalen, Keith Tarr–Whalen, Dr. George Thibault, Newell Thomas, Allan Tobin, Laura Tracy, Dr. Paul Wallace, John Walsh, Simkha Weintraub,

Lynn Whitener, Dr. Karen Wilkerson, Meryl Weinberg, Dr. Marissa Weiss, Tom Weiss, Dr. Jed Weissberg, Herbert Wells, Vera Wells, Ray Werntz, Daphne White, Nancy Whitelaw, Sara Wolch, Elaine Wolfensohn, Judy Woodruff, Mary Wooley, Boe Workman, Simon Wynn, Lou Yaeger, Dr. Paul Zelnik, Dr. Michael Zinner. And twenty-three contributors who declined to be acknowledged to protect their privacy.

National Multiple Sclerosis Society, 246
National Parkinson's Foundation, 246
NeedyMeds, 253
nerve disease resources, 193, 219
New England Journal of Medicine, 20
news media information, 31–32
Nofziger, Ron, 161
nonprofit organizations. *See* voluntary
    and nonprofit organizations
nontreatment alternative, 95–96, 123,
    173–74, 176
nurse practitioners, 226
nurses, xx–xxi, 80, 184, 234–35

O'Connor, Annette, 178
online support. *See* Internet resources
opinion seeking, obsessive, 83, 85. *See
    also* second opinions
optimism and health, 12, 32, 89–91
Ottawa Health Research Institute,
    196–97
outcomes, attaching importance to,
    177–78
out-of-pocket maximum, 142

paid leave benefits, 130
parent's own diagnosis, 54–55
Parkinson's disease resources, 246
Partnership for Prescription Assistance,
    253
Partners Online Specialty
    Consultations, 220
Pashby, Ann, 132, 142
pastoral counselors, 228–29
pathology, 87–88, 92–93
Patient Advocate Foundation, 233, 252
patient advocates, 232–34, 238–39
PatientINFORM, 195
Patient Navigator Act (2005), 236–37
patient navigators, 236–37
patient safety information, 216–17
People Living with Cancer, 243–44
Performance Ratings for Hospitals in
    California, 216
Personal Health Kit, 117–18, 145
personal patient advocate services, 214,
    234

personal research. *See* deliberative
    information-gathering
personal responsibility for choices, xix,
    xx, 174–79
Pew Internet and American Life
    Project, 34
pharmacy benefit plans, 143–44
physical effects of diagnosis, 2, 4, 15,
    155
physical relaxation, 155–56
Physician Data Queries (PDQs), 31,
    198–99
physicians. *See* mental health
    professionals; specialists; *entries
    beginning with "doctor"*
Pinnacle Care International, 234
Pitchon, Mario, 147
Pope, Tara Parker, 207
precertification, 143, 145
primary care providers, 142, 180–81,
    225–26
privacy issues
    and family, 45
    overview, 118–22, 221–23
    at work, 120, 121, 130, 134–35
Privacy Project, 221–22
Privacy Rights Clearinghouse, 222
procedures. *See* treatments and
    procedures
procrastination, 102
prognosis, asking about, 95–96
progress
    author's reflections on, 187–90
    awareness of, 171–72
    examining the possibilities as, 185,
        187
    moving beyond stuck, 180–86
    overcoming emotional upheaval, xx,
        9–10
    trying one thing at a time as, 173
Project Inform National Hotline,
    248–49
provider book, insurance company's,
    145
Psychology Today, 231
public support. *See* government health
    insurance programs; Medicare

Jessie Gruman is the founder and president of the Center for the Advancement of Health, an independent, nonpartisan Washington–based policy institute whose mission is to ensure that people have easy access to the information they need to make good decisions about their health and health care. Dr. Gruman has worked on this same concern in the private sector (AT&T), the public sector (National Cancer Institute), and the voluntary health sector (American Cancer Society).

Dr. Gruman received her undergraduate degree from Vassar College and her Ph.D. in social psychology from Columbia University. She serves on the boards of trustees of the National Health Council, the Public Health Institute, the Sallan Foundation, and the Center for Information Therapy, among others.

A fellow of the Society of Behavioral Medicine and recipient of the Society's awards for distinguished service and "Leadership in Translation of Research to Practice," she has been recognized for outstanding service from the American Psychological Association and recently was honored by Research!America for her leadership in advocacy for health research. She is the recipient of an honorary doctorate in public policy from Carnegie Mellon University and the Presidential Medal of The George Washington University. She served as the executive in residence at Vassar College and is a member of the editorial boards of the *Annals of Family Medicine*, the Society of Behavioral Medicine, the American Psychological Association, the American Psychological Society, and the Council on Foreign Relations.

Dr. Gruman is the author of numerous articles and essays published in the scholarly and public media. She lives in New York and Washington, D.C.

Please visit http://aftershock–book.com for regular updates of the appendices.